HEAI
CRYSTALS

the A – Z guide to 555 gemstones

Michael Gienger

*Translated from the German
by Chinwendu Uzodike*

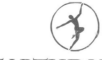

EARTHDANCER

A FINDHORN PRESS IMPRINT

Publisher's note

The information in this volume has been compiled according to the best of our knowledge and belief, and the healing properties of the crystals have been tested many times over. Bearing in mind that different people react in different ways, neither the publisher nor the author can guarantee the effectiveness or safety of use in individual cases. In the case of serious health problems, please consult your doctor or naturopath.

2nd (revised) edition 2014
First edition published in 2005 by Earthdancer GmbH,
reprinted: 2006, 2007, 2009, 2010, 2011, 2012

Healing Crystals – Michael Gienger, With photos by Ines Blersch
Published by Earthdancer GmbH, an Imprint of: Findhorn Press Ltd, 117-121 High Street, Forres, IV36 1AB, Scotland. www.earthdancer.co.uk, www.findhornpress.com

This English edition © 2014 Earthdancer GmbH
English translation © 2014 Chinwendu Uzodike
Editing of the translated text by JMS Books LLP, www.jmswords.com

Originally published in German as *Heilsteine, 555 Steine von A–Z*

World copyright
© 2013 Neue Erde GmbH, Saarbruecken, Germany
Original German text copyright
© 2013 Michael Gienger

Cover photography: Ines Blersch
Cover and book design: Dragon Design UK
Typeset in News Gothic
Printed and bound in China

ISBN 978-1-84409-647-3

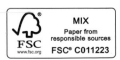

MIX
Paper from
responsible sources
FSC® C011223
www.fsc.org

The clear and comprehensive guide to the healing power of crystals

Work on this guide started in 1993 and the first edition was published in 2003; since then, it has sold more than 500,000 copies in German alone and been translated into seven other languages. Now, in 2013, Michael Gienger presents this revised and extended edition, prompted by new findings in mineralogy as well as new experiences and research results in the field of gem therapy.

It would not have been possible to compile this compact but comprehensive guide without the professional advice of the geologist Dr. Andreas Stucki and the mineralogist Bernhard Bruder, as well as the support of many naturopaths, doctors and gemstone consultants. Heartfelt thanks go to all those who have contributed to making this work a reality! In this completely revised edition, Michael Gienger describes the specific healing properties of 555 individual crystals in a clear and concise form that makes this pocket guide invaluable.

The guide is intended for all those who seek a simple and reliable source of information on healing crystals:

- For anyone who wishes to learn about the healing properties of crystals.

- For naturopaths, doctors and gemstone consultants, as an up-to-date reference guide to healing crystals.

- For those who work with or deal in crystals, as an important update on the latest developments in the field of gem remedy.

In a word: a guide for anyone who relates to crystals. So take a look...

How to use this guide

The guide presents and defines the mineralogy and healing effects of crystals in common use, offering concise information on their basic properties. For further information, consult the indicated bibliography as needed. Terms used in the guide are as follows:

Title: the title of each entry gives the name or names of the illustrated crystal. In addition to the mineralogical name, the common or trade name is also used where relevant to define or describe the crystal in question. The scientifically recognised mineralogical names are printed in black, while common names are printed in blue. The titles serve as a suggestion to both gemstone dealers and interested readers of the correct and clear designation of the crystals.

Mineralogy: this gives a brief definition of the mineral with respect to the mineralogy, especially its crystalline structure and nature of formation ('prim.' = molten magma formation, 'sec.' = formation through disintegration and deposits, 'tert.' = metamorphic formation under heat and pressure).* In addition to the visible colour, these details are very important for the healing effect and application of a crystal. For further information on their significance, see Michael Gienger's book *Crystal Power, Crystal Healing* (Cassell, London, 1998).

Indications: this gives information on the most important healing effects and areas of activity of each crystal, in particular the main properties that characterise the crystal and distinguish it from crystals with similar properties. Other healing effects can be found in the indicated bibliography.

(SP) refers to the 'spirit' or 'spiritual aspect', the innate nature of a person including his or her important intentions, aims and focus in life; (S) refers to the 'soul' or the 'subconscious', including temperament, emotions, intuitive perceptions, dreams, psychological experiences, habits and unconscious reactions; (M) refers to 'mind' or 'mental aspects', including ideas, values, convictions, views as well as the manner of thinking and conscious action; (B) refers to the 'body' or 'physical aspect', the human organism as a whole with its senses, organs and functions.

Defining these four aspects clearly differentiates what can be influenced, enhanced, changed or cured with the help of the crystals.

---

* **Abbreviations:**	tert. = tertiary	trig. = trigonal	mon. = monoclinic
prim. = primary	cub. = cubic	tetr. = tetragonal	tric. = triclinic
sec. = secondary	hex. = hexagonal	rhom. = rhombic	am. = amorphous

Bib.: this refers to comprehensive literature in which the crystal in question, or at least crystals of the same kind or family, is described. The numbers 1 to 21 refer to the bibliography on page 123.

Rarity: this gives an estimate of the availability of the crystal in question. Naturally, this is often subject to variation depending on which crystals are collected or mined in which mines or discovery sites at any point in time. As a result, these estimates are never 'absolute' – they are only intended to give a clue as to the chances of finding a desired crystal in the shops in the foreseeable future. Also, the availability of a crystal is not always linked to how rare or common it is. Rare crystals that are well known are sometimes more readily available than more common but less known ones. The availability has been individually classified as follows:

Common: means it has been continuously available in large quantities over a long period of time and cut into different forms and shapes. No scarcity of the common shapes or forms is anticipated in the foreseeable future.

Readily available: means it is available most of the time. No major scarcities of particular forms are expected in the future.

Not always available: means not always obtainable. Sometimes there is a scarcity or just a few forms are available in limited quantities. The reserves fluctuate or are limited.

Scarce: means hardly available. There is a frequent scarcity over long periods of time. It is sometimes only available in very few forms. Reserves are very limited.

Rare: means extremely scarce and obtainable only at specific times. For such crystals there is only a minimal reserve, or the known discovery sites are already exhausted or no longer accessible.

◯ This little tick box enables you to make a note of the crystals you have – giving you an overview of crystals in your collection, first aid kit, experiment kit or therapy repertoire.

Abalone (Paua shell, Mother-of-pearl)
Mineralogy: coloured shell (Aragonite, rhom., sec.)
Indications: (SP) cheerfulness, security, protection (S) helps overcome despondency, insecurity and disappointment (M) ensures careful dealing with oneself and others (B) ameliorates irritation and inflammations of skin, mucous membrane and sensory organs.
Bib.: 2 | 4 | 6 | 8   **Rarity:** common ○

Actinolite
Mineralogy: chain silicate of the Amphibole group (mon., tert.)
Indications: (SP) straightforwardness, realignment, determination (S) promotes self-esteem and inner balance (M) helps pursue personal aims with determination (B) stimulates activity of the liver and kidney as well as all building-up and growth processes.
Bib.: 1 | 2 | 4–8   **Rarity:** not always available

Actinolite Quartz
Mineralogy: actinolite in quartz crystal (mon./trig., prim./tert.)
Indications: (SP) realignment, awareness, course correction (S) enhances sense of right timing (M) aids in overcoming weaknesses and mistakes (B) stimulates the liver and kidneys as well as metabolism; detoxification and excretion.
Bib.: 1 | 2–6 | 8   **Rarity:** scarce

Aegirine
Mineralogy: chain silicate of the pyroxene group (mon., prim.)
Indications: (SP) sincerity, virtue (S) promotes self-respect, helpful with relationship problems, separation or grief (M) focusing on major goals (B) helps with backache and pains, good for nerves, muscles, bones and hormonal glands.
Bib.: 4 | 6 | 8 | 9   **Rarity:** scarce ○

Aegirine-Augite in Matrix
Mineralogy: chain silicate of the pyroxene group (mon., prim.)
Indications: (SP) posture; perseverance (S) encourages patience, helps maintain composure in difficult situations (M) for work requiring patience (mental and physical) (B) enhances digestion, activity of the intestine, kidneys, and hormonal glands; ameliorates pain.
Bib.: 4 | 6   **Rarity:** scarce ○

Agate

Mineralogy: banded quartz (SiO_2, trig., prim./sec.)

Indications: (SP) stability, composure, maturity (S) protection, warmth, security (M) sense of reality, pragmatic thinking, easy resolution of problems (B) for the eyes, hollow organs (like the stomach, intestines etc.), blood vessels and skin. Protective stone in pregnancy.

Bib.: 1–7 | 11 | 13 | 14 | 16 | 18 | 19   **Rarity:** common ○

Agate 'with bladder-like markings'

Mineralogy: agate with bladder-like markings (trig., prim./sec.)

Indications: (SP) self-control, letting go, inner calm (S) setting boundaries, relaxation (M) helps to implement ideas or projects resolutely (B) for bladder problems, especially infections, urinary retention, incontinence and prostate.

Bib.: 1–6 | 8 | 10 | 13 | 14 | 16 | 18   **Rarity:** readily available

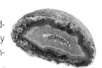

Agate 'Brecciated Agate'

Mineralogy: tectonically deformed agate (trig., prim.)

Indications: (SP) self-assurance (S) makes untouchable in the face of destructive forces (M) helps to correct grave mistakes and put things in order (B) for wound healing and attenuation of scars in cases of diaphragmatic and inguinal hernia and bone fractures.

Bib.: 2 | 4 | 6 | 8   **Rarity:** rare ○

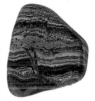

Agate 'with cell-like markings'

Mineralogy: agate with cell/tissue-type markings (trig., prim.)

Indications: (SP) versatility, regeneration (S) revives dazed frame of mind (M) enhances concentration on the essential (B) for tissues, metabolism, immune system; helps with infections and skin diseases.

Bib.: 2–5 | 13 | 14   **Rarity:** not always available ○

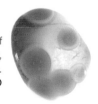

Agate 'Crazy Lace'

Mineralogy: agate with twisting and turning bands (trig., prim.)

Indications: (SP) dexterity, mental agility, joie de vivre (S) makes life more intensive, promotes curiosity (M) helps break the routine of sticking to the habitual (B) very effective against infections, insect bites, varicose veins, haemorrhoids and venous ulcers.

Bib.: 2–6 | 8 | 13 | 14 | 17   **Rarity:** readily available

Agate 'Crystal Agate'

Mineralogy: agate with clear quartz (trig., prim./sec.)
Indications: (SP) renewal of self-concept (S) helps deal with experiences and awakens suppressed memories (M) promotes the recognition of logical interconnections (B) good for the eyes, stomach, intestine and bladder, good protective stone in pregnancy.
Bib.: 1 | 2 | 4   **Rarity:** not always available

Agate 'Dendritic Agate'

Mineralogy: agate with fern-like manganese markings (trig., prim./sec.)
Indications: (SP) integrity, purification (S) helps overcome emotional boundary violations and emotional burdens (M) lends ability to examine and resolve unpleasant issues (B) for tissue detoxification in problems of the skin, mucous membrane, lungs and intestine.
Bib.: 1–6 | 8   **Rarity:** not always available

Agate 'Agate with escape tube'

Mineralogy: agate with outlet channels (trig., prim./sec.)
Indications: (SP) encounter, trust (S) instils the need to fulfil one's needs, helps to deal with pressure (M) makes one open to new impulses, fantasy and creativity (B) fortifies the urinary tract, bladder, prostate gland and genital organs, alleviates pressure-induced discomforts.
Bib.: 4   **Rarity:** scarce

Agate 'Eye Agate'

Mineralogy: agate with eye-shaped markings (trig., prim./sec.)
Indications: (SP) interest, resistance, protection (S) perseverance, also in the face of nightmares (M) helps face facts (B) for inflammation of the eyes, problems of the conjunctiva or retina, glaucoma, blood vessels and prostate.
Bib.: 1–6 | 8 | 10 | 13 | 14 | 16 | 18   **Rarity:** readily available ○

Agate 'Fire Agate'

Mineralogy: agate with iridescent hematite layers (trig., prim.)
Indications: (SP) initiative, commitment (S) cheerfulness, contentment (M) vigour, positive thinking, understanding experiences (B) for excretion, problems of the intestine, especially flatulence, diarrhoea, constipation, (chronic) inflammation.
Bib.: 2–6 | 8 | 11 | 13 | 14   **Rarity:** scarce

Agate 'Flame Agate'
Mineralogy: agate with flame markings (trig., prim./sec.)
Indications: (SP) protection and sensibility **(S)** promotes friendliness and objectivity, helps cope with emotional wounds **(M)** makes attentive and prompts one to seize opportunities **(B)** strengthens sensory organs, tissues covering organs and hollow organs.
Bib.: 2 | 4 | 6 | 8   **Rarity:** readily available

Agate 'Fortification Agate'
Mineralogy: agate with fortification-like markings (trig., prim./sec.)
Indications: (SP) steadfastness, stability **(S)** enhances protection, security and endurance **(M)** promotes precision and perfection **(B)** stabilises blood circulation, helps with dizziness and sensitivity to weather changes, strengthens spleen, stomach, pancreas, intestine, bladder.
Bib.: 2–6 | 8 | 12   **Rarity:** scarce

Agate 'with inflammation markings'
Mineralogy: agate with natural pink colour (trig., prim./sec.)
Indications: (SP) transformation, consolation, appeasement **(S)** renewed confidence in unpleasant situations **(M)** careful mastering of difficulties **(B)** for inflammation of all organs or tissues; enhances perspiration during fever.
Bib.: 1–6 | 8 | 10 | 13 | 14 | 16 | 18 **Rarity:** not always available ○

Agate 'Lace Agate'
Mineralogy: agate with twisting and turning bands (trig., prim.)
Indications: (SP) elegance, mental agility, dynamism **(S)** liveliness, variety **(M)** flexibility in thinking and acting **(B)** promotes tissue metabolism, very effective against infections, insect bites, varicose veins, haemorrhoids and venous ulcers.
Bib.: 2–6 | 8 | 13 | 14 | 17   **Rarity:** readily available

Agate 'Lamellae Agate'
Mineralogy: agate with prominent lamellae (trig., prim./sec.)
Indications: (SP) promotes introspection, balance between activity and rest **(S)** resistance against undesired influences **(M)** promotes an eye for detail and concentration on the essential **(B)** good for equilibrium, nerves, senses, skin, lungs, large intestine and bladder.
Bib.: 4   **Rarity:** not always available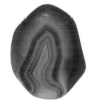

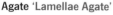
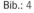

Agate 'Layered Agate', 'Banded Agate'
Mineralogy: agate with band-like layers (trig., prim./sec.)
Indications: **(SP)** steadfastness and unity **(S)** protection, security, moral stability **(M)** for pragmatic planning in thinking and actions **(B)** for the intestine and digestion; improves elasticity of blood vessel walls and prevents varicose veins.
Bib.: 1–6 | 8 | 10 | 13 | 14 | 16 | 18   **Rarity:** readily available

Agate 'Petrified Wood Agate'
Mineralogy: agate in petrified wood (trig., sec.)
Indications: **(SP)** composure and modesty **(S)** for deep-rooted inner peace, helps cope with burdens **(M)** makes down-to-earth, sober and realistic **(B)** enhances digestion, strengthens the connective tissues, calms the nerves and helps with neurovegetative dystonia.
Bib.: 4   **Rarity:** scarce ○

Agate, pink 'Apricot Agate'
Mineralogy: agate, predominantly pink coloured (trig., prim./sec.)
Indications: **(SP)** incentive, compassion **(S)** steadfastness, protection and safety **(M)** helps to deal positively with difficult assignments **(B)** for inflammation; activates absorption of nutrients in the intestine and also stimulates metabolism and blood circulation.
Bib.: 2–6 | 8 | 11 | 13 | 14   **Rarity:** not always available ∅

Agate, red 'Blood Agate'
Mineralogy: agate with a natural red colour (trig., prim./sec.)
Indications: **(SP)** strength, stability, increases stamina **(S)** perseverance and strength generated from inner balance **(M)** development and conscious usage of personal abilities **(B)** fortifies stomach, intestine and blood vessels, enhances circulation and blood-flow.
Bib.: 1–6 | 8 | 11 | 13 | 14   **Rarity:** not always available ∅

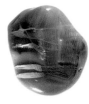

Agate 'with scar images'
Mineralogy: agate with scar-like images (trig., prim./sec.)
Indications: **(SP)** makes amends, eases burdens **(S)** overcomes past injuries **(M)** helps to cope positively with stress and strain **(B)** improves skin and tissue metabolism, enhances wound healing, and reduces scar formation.
Bib.: 2 | 3 | 4 | 5   **Rarity:** not always available ○

Agate 'with skin-like image'
Mineralogy: agate, similar to layers of the skin (trig., prim./sec.)
Indications: (SP) contact, setting boundaries **(S)** stability and perseverance **(M)** constructive reflection **(B)** regulates, builds up, detoxifies the skin, for rashes, inflammations, fungal infections, as well as dry, chapped or impure skin.
Bib.: 1–6 | 8 | 13 | 14 | 16 | 18   **Rarity:** readily available

Agate 'Snakeskin Agate' (Chalcedony)
Mineralogy: agate, similar to the skin of a snake (trig., sec.)
Indications: (SP) clarification, communication **(S)** calms agitated emotions **(M)** for realistic thinking and well-considered actions **(B)** good for the brain, metabolism, lymph and body fluids, decongests mucous and ameliorates allergies.
Bib.: 2 | 4 | 6 | 8   **Rarity:** scarce

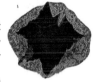

Agate 'Star Agate'
Mineralogy: Star-like agate in lithophysa (trig., prim.)
Indications: (SP) consciousness, alertness, maturity **(S)** confident self-expression and emotional stability **(M)** promotes a good understanding and recognition of interconnections **(B)** enhances digestion, the senses, nerves, spinal cord, brain, immune system and hormone balance.
Bib.: 2 | 4–6 | 8   **Rarity:** not always available ○

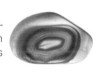

Agate 'with stomach-like markings'
Mineralogy: agate with stomach like markings (trig., prim./sec.)
Indications: (SP) life experience, work **(S)** enhances absorption of impressions and experiences **(M)** promotes learning and sober reflection **(B)** for digestion and metabolism, for stomach and intestine problems e.g. nausea or gastritis.
Bib.: 1–6 | 10 | 13 | 14 | 16 | 18   **Rarity:** readily available ○

Agate 'Thunderegg', 'Amulet stone'
Mineralogy: agate in a rhyolite or porphyritic nodule (trig., prim.)
Indications: (SP) helps with awakening one's potential **(S)** for conserving one's energy, good perceptive faculty **(M)** for fulfilling one's needs, resolving difficult problems **(B)** for the stomach, pancreas, intestine, liver, nerves, spinal cord, brain, immune system and hormone balance.
Bib.: 2–6 | 8   **Rarity:** not always available ○

Agate 'Tubular Agate'
Mineralogy: agate with tube-like inclusions (trig., prim./sec.)
Indications: (SP) unfolding, progress (S) tenacity, acceptance of the inevitable (M) insight, reconsider views (B) promotes activity of the glands and metabolism; very effective for prostate, bladder and digestive problems; aids sexual endeavours.
Bib.: 2 | 4 | 6   **Rarity:** scarce ○

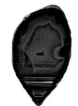

Agate 'Uruguay Agate'
Mineralogy: agate with horizontal layers (trig., prim./sec.)
Indications: (SP) conserving one's energy (S) clarifies agitated emotions, brings inner balance, helps with stress (M) enhances resolution of difficulties and disputes (B) good for the intestine, connective tissue and skin, helps with water blisters and swellings.
Bib.: 2 | 4 | 6 | 8   **Rarity:** not always available ○

Agate 'with uterus-shaped markings'
Mineralogy: agate with uterus-shaped markings (trig., prim./sec.)
Indications: (SP) growth, development, blossoming (S) instils deep security when homesick or lonely (M) mindfulness (B) for inflammation of the uterus, menstrual pain, pregnancy and normalisation after childbirth.
Bib.: 1–6 | 10 | 13 | 14 | 16 | 18   **Rarity:** readily available ○

Agate 'Water Agate', 'Enhydro'
Mineralogy: agate nodule filled with water (trig., prim./sec.)
Indications: (SP) growth, protection, development (S) instils deep security and enhances inner peace, promotes empathy (M) fortifies solicitude and openness (B) protective stone in pregnancy; regulates water and hormone balance.
Bib.: 1–6 | 8 | 13 | 14   **Rarity:** scarce ○

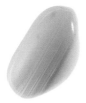

Agate, white 'Peace Agate'
Mineralogy: colourless, white agate (trig., prim./sec.)
Indications: (SP) calm, peace, self-confidence (S), strengthens inner composure, for kindness, sincerity and light-heartedness (M) promotes tolerance and understanding (B) for the eyes, brain, skin, lymph and tissues; protective stone in pregnancy.
Bib.: 2 | 4–6 | 8   **Rarity:** readily available ○

Agate, white/black 'Zebra Agate'
Mineralogy: agate with black/white stripes (trig., prim./sec.)
Indications: (SP) reformation, reflection, maturity **(S)** promotes objectivity and straightforwardness **(M)** enhances meticulousness; for objective and rational ordering of one's life **(B)** improves activity of motor nerves, sense of hearing and balance.
Bib.: 2 | 4–6 | 8 **Rarity:** not always available

Agatised Coral
Mineralogy: fossilised corals (lime or quartz, trig., sec.)
Indications: (SP) self-expression, hospitality **(S)** eases fear as well as emotional and social strain **(M)** promotes ability to communicate, team spirit and synergy in partnership **(B)** helps with breathing difficulties, cramped bronchial tubes and cough.
Bib.: 2 | 4 | 6 | 8 | 17 **Rarity:** not always available ○

Alabaster (Gypsum)
Mineralogy: fine crystalline calcium sulphate (mon., sec.)
Indications: (SP) stability, self-control, setting boundaries **(S)** helps set boundaries and stabilise labile psychic state, protects in cases of hypersensitivity **(M)** conscious recognition of old patterns **(B)** loosens up hardened muscles and firms up tissues, cartilage and bones.
Bib.: 2 | 4–6 | 16 | 17 **Rarity:** readily available ○

Alabaster orange (Gypsum)
Mineralogy: fine crystalline, ferruginous gypsum (mon., sec.)
Indications: (SP) goodwill, unity **(S)** inner composure and integration of experiences **(M)** reflection on oneself and the tasks at hand **(B)** helps with chronic state of debility and strengthens muscles, tendons, ligaments and joints.
Bib.: 2 | 4–6 | 16 | 17 **Rarity:** readily available ○

Alabaster Engelberg (Gypsum)
Mineralogy: alabaster nodule from Leonberg (mon., sec.)
Indications: (SP) self-awareness, setting boundaries **(S)** for calm and relaxation, helps overcome old habits, intensifies dreams **(M)** helps establish priorities **(B)** for restful sleep, improves well-being, alleviates pain and releases tension.
Bib.: 2 | 4–6 | 8 **Rarity:** scarce

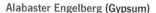

Albite, light-blue (Feldspar)

Mineralogy: lead-containing sodium feldspar (lattice silicate, tric., prim.)
Indications: (SP) self-acceptance, self-acknowledgement (S) balance between inner needs and external reality (M) helps to better assess the true value and importance of many things (B) for flexible muscles and confident use of motor skills, strengthens the kidneys and bladder.
Bib.: 2 | 4 | 6 | 8   **Rarity:** not always available

Albite, white (Feldspar)

Mineralogy: sodium feldspar (lattice silicate, tric., prim./tert.)
Indications: (SP) intuitive perception, broadens horizons (S) brings relief, opening and wideness (M) improves perceptive faculty, helps recognise new perspectives in life (B) eases breathing, good for the eyes, ears, pliable tissues and healthy skin.
Bib.: 2 | 4 | 6 | 8   **Rarity:** scarce

Alexandrite (Chrysoberyl)

Mineralogy: chromium-containing chrysoberyl (rhom., tert.)
Indications: (SP) clairvoyance and willpower (S) intensifies dreams and perception of emotions (M) promotes power of imagination, willingness to take risks and perception of inner voice (B) for disorders of the nerves and senses; ameliorates inflammations, boosts the liver.
Bib.: 1 | 2 | 4 | 6 | 8 | 19   **Rarity:** rare

Allalin Gabbro

Mineralogy: eclogite-facies metagabbro (largely mon., tert.)
Indications: (SP) success through calm tenacity (S) lends patience, perseverance and self-confidence (M) makes decision-making easier (B) enhances the liver and kidneys as well as all regeneration, growth and anabolic processes in the body.
Bib.: 4   **Rarity:** not always available

Almandine (Garnet)

Mineralogy: iron aluminium island silicate (cub., tert.)
Indications: (SP) increases powers of resistance (S) fortifies willpower and helps live one's sexuality (M) aids insight and helps achieve one's ideas against great resistance (B) activates and stimulates circulation, blood-building and metabolism.
Bib.: 1–14 | 16 | 17 | 19   **Rarity:** readily available

Alunite (Alum Stone)
Mineralogy: potassium aluminium sulphate (trig., prim./sec.)
Indications: (SP) comfort, modesty (S) settles discords, disperses fear and guilty conscience (M) encourages frugality and being reserved (B) helps in cases of chronic inflammation, eczema and rashes as well as radiation damage.
Bib.: 2 | 4 | 6 | 8   Rarity: not always available

Amazonite (Feldspar)
Mineralogy: green feldspar containing lead (tric./mon., prim.)
Indications: (SP) determination of one's destiny (S) emotional balance (M) harmonious interaction of intellect and intuition (B) regulates metabolic disorders (liver); harmonises the brain, vegetative nervous system, internal organs; facilitates childbirth.
Bib.: 1 | 2 | 4–8 | 10 | 11 | 13 | 14 | 17   Rarity: readily available

Amber, black
Mineralogy: black fossiliferous resin (organic, am., sec.)
Indications: (SP) for farewell, letting-go (S) helps with worries and fear, supports hospice work (M) focuses attention on concrete goals (B) prevents infections, fortifies the feet and back muscles, protects the spine.
Bib.: 4 | 6 | 8 | 19 | 20   Rarity: scarce

Amber, blue
Mineralogy: yellowish blue fossiliferous resin (organic, am., sec.)
Indications: (SP) wisdom, understanding (S) lends willingness to help and enables living in harmony with others (M) helps maintain one's standpoint while being receptive to that of others (B) good for the nerves, respiratory tract, thyroid gland and hormone system.
Bib.: 4 | 19 | 20   Rarity: rare

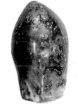

Amber, brown
Mineralogy: brown fossiliferous resin (organic, am., sec.)
Indications: (SP) for strength, blossoming (S) dissipates anger, aggression, dissatisfaction, envy, vengefulness and jealousy (M) reduces selfishness and helps expend energy meaningfully (B) good for the stomach, intestine and bladder, helps with pains of the lower back.
Bib.: 1–14 | 16 | 17 | 19 | 20   Rarity: readily available

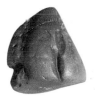

Amber, red

Mineralogy: red fossiliferous resin (organic, am., sec.)
Indications: (SP) love and bravery **(S)** helps keep one's nature strong and unharmed **(M)** promotes determination, courage and willpower **(B)** eases heart problems, regulates blood pressure and helps with ailments of the male genitals.

Bib.: 4 | 19 | 20   **Rarity:** scarce ○

Amber, white

Mineralogy: white fossiliferous resin (organic, am., sec.)
Indications: (SP) kindness and joy **(S)** makes carefree, brings well-being and helps realign extremes **(M)** promotes traditional ties and brings success **(B)** good for the brain, nerves, heart, lymph and hormone system, helps with hoarseness and sore throat.

Bib.: 4–6 | 8 | 19 | 20   **Rarity:** not always available ◑

Amber, yellow

Mineralogy: yellow fossiliferous resin (organic, am., sec.)
Indications: (SP) makes carefree **(S)** for cheerfulness and trust **(M)** strengthens belief in oneself **(B)** good for the stomach, spleen, pancreas, gallbladder, liver, joints, skin, mucous membranes, glands and intestine; aids teething, helps with allergies, rheumatism and diabetes.

Bib.: 1–14 | 16 | 17 | 19 | 20   **Rarity:** readily available ◑

Amethyst, dark purple (Quartz)

Mineralogy: dark violet crystal quartz (trig., sec.)
Indications: (SP) alertness, impartiality, inner peace **(S)** helps overcome pain, grief and losses **(M)** awareness, sense of judgement, constructive thinking and acting **(B)** good for the skin; alleviates pain and tension and lowers high blood pressure.

Bib.: 1–7 | 10 | 11 | 13 | 14 | 16–19 | 21 **Rarity:** readily available ○

Amethyst, light purple (Quartz)

Mineralogy: light violet crystal quartz (trig., sec.)
Indications: (SP) peace, spirituality, clarification, meditation **(S)** for intuition, good clear dreams, improves fitful sleep **(M)** enhances conscious perception and understanding experiences **(B)** relieves headaches, good for the lungs, skin and nerves.

Bib.: 1–7 | 10 | 11 | 13 | 14 | 16–19 | 21   **Rarity:** common ◑

Amethyst, very dark purple (Quartz)

Mineralogy: very dark violet crystal quartz (trig., prim.)

Indications: (SP) uprightness, impartiality (S) willpower, helps overcome pain, grief and losses (M) improves concentration, helps ward off external influences (B) alleviates pain, bruises and swellings, diarrhoea.

Bib.: 1–8 | 11 | 13 | 14   Rarity: scarce ○

Amethyst Quartz 'Chevron Amethyst' (Quartz)

Mineralogy: violet/white striped crystal quartz (trig., prim.)

Indications: (SP) sobriety, purity, composure, calm (S) peps up in cases of perpetual tiredness, resolves persistent anxiety (M) helps overcome habitual tendencies and addictions (B) good for the lungs, large intestine and skin; alleviates itching and sunburn.

Bib.: 1–7 | 11 | 13 | 14 | 17   Rarity: common ∅

Amethyst with Chalcedony (Quartz)

Mineralogy: amethyst with chalcedony stripes (trig., sec.)

Indications: (SP) reconciliation, peace, kindness (S) promotes feelings of happiness and universal love (M) helps trigger self-reconciliation and reconciliation between individuals (B) cleanses body fluids and harmonises the whole organism.

Bib.: 4 | 6 | 8   Rarity: scarce ∅

Ametrine (Quartz)

Mineralogy: yellow/violet crystal quartz (trig., prim./sec./tert.)

Indications: (SP) cheerful composure, a fulfilled existence (S) optimism, joie de vivre, feeling of well-being (M) helps retain creativity and dynamism in the face of all challenges (B) balances out body tension, harmonises the vegetative nervous system and body metabolism.

Bib.: 1 | 2 | 4–6 | 8 | 9 | 14 | 17 | 19   Rarity: scarce ○

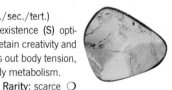

Ammolite (Korite, Calcentine)

Mineralogy: ammonite shell made of aragonite (rhom., sec.)

Indications: (SP) harmony, dignity, splendour (S) for sense of beauty, seductive charm, charisma (M) awakens interest in mysteries, releases mental obsessions (B) normalises cell metabolism, energy output, heartbeat and fortifies the heart.

Bib.: 4 | 6 | 8   Rarity: rare ○

Amphibolite
Mineralogy: hornblende with feldspar (mon./tric., tert.)
Indications: (SP) balanced nature, equanimity (S) brings calm, helps overcome dissatisfaction and frustration (M) lends vigour and helps let go of expectations (B) good for the autonomic nervous system, digestion, kidneys, ears, vocal cords and larynx.
Bib.: 4 | 6   **Rarity:** not always available ○

Andalusite
Mineralogy: aluminium island silicate (rhom., tert.)
Indications: (SP) self-recognition, discovery of personal vocation (S) promotes self-confidence and generosity (M) helps to think big and be realistic at the same time (B) enhances de-acidification, good for stomach and intestine problems; has a strengthening effect.
Bib.: 2 | 4 | 6 | 8   **Rarity:** not always available ◑

Andradite (Garnet)
Mineralogy: calcium iron island silicate (cub., tert.)
Indications: (SP) willpower, orientation (S) for intuition, safety and trust (M) enhances creativity, shrewdness and flexibility (B) stimulates the liver and blood-building; improves vitality, mobility and fitness; helps with absence of menstruation.
Bib.: 1 | 2 | 4 | 6 | 8 | 16 | 19   **Rarity:** scarce ○

Anhydrite, blue (Angelite)
Mineralogy: anhydrous calcium sulphate (rhom., sec.)
Indications: (SP) stability, stamina (S) helps withstand extreme psychic strain and overcome insecurity (M) ends fruitless brooding and helps give up obsessions (B) stimulates kidney function, water balance and reduction of oedema.
Bib.: 2 | 4 | 6 | 8   **Rarity:** not always available ○

Anhydrite, violet
Mineralogy: anhydrous calcium sulphate (rhom., sec.)
Indications: (SP) grounding, protection, moral stability (S) helps overcome feelings of guilt and emotional shock (M) aids taking control of one's life (B) promotes detoxification, strengthens the kidneys, bladder and elasticity of the bones.
Bib.: 2 | 4 | 6 | 8   **Rarity:** not always available ◑

Anthophyllite

Mineralogy: anthophyllite/staurolite rock (rhom., tert.)

Indications: **(SP)** self-esteem, acknowledgement **(S)** releases stress and self-imposed pressure **(M)** helps create and maintain space for personal interest **(B)** helps with nervous diseases as well as with problems of the kidneys and ears.

Bib.: 2 | 4–6 | 8 | 17 **Rarity:** scarce ○

Antimonite

Mineralogy: dark grey antimonite sulphide (rhom., tert.)

Indications: **(SP)** harmonises personal interests with higher ideals **(S)** helps give up negative habits **(M)** helps overcome limiting views **(B)** helps with problems of the digestive tract (stomach), gum and skin (peeling).

Bib.: 1–6 | 8 | 9 | 14 **Rarity:** not always available ⌀

Apatite, black

Mineralogy: black calcium phosphate (hex., prim./tert.)

Indications: **(SP)** independence **(S)** promotes self-conquest and boosts performance **(M)** helps put one's energy to good use **(B)** helps with ailments resulting from incessant strain like tinnitus, high blood pressure, irritable bowel, kidney and bladder problems.

Bib.: 1–6 | 8 | 9 | 13 | 14 **Rarity:** scarce ⌀

Apatite, blue

Mineralogy: blue calcium phosphate (hex., prim./tert.)

Indications: **(SP)** motivation **(S)** stabilises, helps combat listlessness after over-exertion **(M)** promotes independence and ambitiousness **(B)** builds up, de-acidifies and helps with rickets, arthrosis, osteoporosis and the healing of fractures.

Bib.: 1–8 | 10 | 11 | 13 | 14 | 17 **Rarity:** readily available ⌀

Apatite, green

Mineralogy: green calcium phosphate (hex., prim./tert.)

Indications: **(SP)** sociable **(S)** livens up, helps combat listlessness after over-exertion **(M)** helps live life full of variety **(B)** builds up, de-acidifies, enhances formation of cartilage, bones and teething, also helps with fractures.

Bib.: 1–6 | 8–10 | 13 | 14 **Rarity:** not always available ⌀

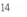

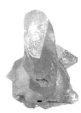

Apatite, pink

Mineralogy: pink calcium phosphate (hex., prim./tert.)
Indications: (SP) tactful (S) makes cheerful and livens up one's life (M) lends understanding and tolerance for oneself and others (B) helps with sensitivity to physical contact, overwrought nerves, metabolic disorders and heart problems caused by fatigue.
Bib.: 1–6 | 8 | 9 | 13 | 14   **Rarity:** scarce ○

Apatite, red

Mineralogy: red calcium phosphate (hex., prim./tert.)
Indications: (SP) makes active and energetic (S) reinvigorates after over-exertion, sexually stimulates, helps with impotence (M) awakens interest in life (B) strengthens the muscles and muscle performance, stimulates blood circulation, helps with bone, cartilage and joint problems.
Bib.: 1–6 | 8 | 9 | 13 | 14   **Rarity:** scarce ○

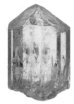

Apatite, yellow

Mineralogy: yellow calcium phosphate (hex., prim./tert.)
Indications: (SP) drive (S) makes extrovert, invigorates and livens up, helps out of state of apathy (M) promotes optimism and hopefulness (B) stimulates appetite; mobilises energy reserves; improves posture; helps with problems of the bones, cartilage and joints.
Bib.: 1–6 | 8–10 | 13 | 14   **Rarity:** scarce ⬿

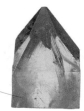

Apophyllite, colourless

Mineralogy: water-containing sheet silicate (tetr., sec.)
Indications: (SP) openness, frankness (S) helps overcome insecurity and openly show real nature (M) helps relinquish anxious tendencies and thought patterns (B) helps with problems of the skin, mucous membrane and respiratory tract, allergies and asthma.
Bib.: 1–8 | 11–14   **Rarity:** readily available ○

Apophyllite, green

Mineralogy: water-containing sheet silicate (tetr., sec.)
Indications: (SP) liberation, sincerity (S) helps with fear, pressure and feeling of oppression, releases withheld emotions (M) offers a moment of respite after great exertion (B) helps with problems of the nerves, skin and respiratory tract, allergies and asthma.
Bib.: 1–8 | 11–14   **Rarity:** scarce ○

Aquamarine (Beryl)

Mineralogy: iron-containing beryl, blue to green (hex., prim.)
Indications: (SP) farsightedness, foresight (S) bestows perseverance, discipline, light-heartedness (M) clears up confusion, helps to bring unfinished business to a conclusion (B) helps with allergies, hay fever, problems of the eyes, respiratory tract, thyroid gland and bladder.
Bib.: 1–11 | 13 | 14 | 16–19   Rarity: readily available

Aragonite, blue

Mineralogy: blue calcium carbonate (rhom., sec.)
Indications: (SP) harmonious development (S) helps maintain inner balance (M) stimulates a pleasurable and cheerful shaping of one's life (B) anti-inflammatory, cooling and cramp-releasing effect, helps with joint injuries, arthritis and itching.
Bib.: 2–9 | 11 | 14 | 17   Rarity: not always available ○

Aragonite, brown

Mineralogy: brown calcium carbonate (rhom., sec.)
Indications: (SP) progressive development (S) strengthens when over-taxed and under strain (M) enables proper assessment and handling of situations (B) enhances digestion, good for the teeth, bones, cartilage, discs, meniscus (knee) and helps with rheumatism.
Bib.: 2–9 | 11 | 14 | 17   Rarity: not always available ⌀

Aragonite, crystalline

Mineralogy: crystalline calcium carbonate (rhom., sec.)
Indications: (SP) meaningful development (S) aids when overwhelmed by too many impressions and tasks (M) motivates orientation towards the feasible and essential (B) promotes tooth development, eases teething, good for the discs and meniscus (knee).
Bib.: 1–9 | 11 | 14 | 17   Rarity: not always available ⌀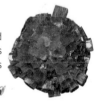

Aragonite, white

Mineralogy: white calcium carbonate (rhom., sec.)
Indications: (SP) stable development (S) combats oversensitivity, stabilises exceedingly fast developments (M) promotes concentration, calms erratic behaviour (B) improves nervous spasms, strengthens muscles, bones, discs, immune system and improves digestion.
Bib.: 1–9 | 11 | 14 | 17   Rarity: not always available ○

Aragonite-Calcite, banded

Mineralogy: calcium carbonate (rhom./trig., sec.)
Indications: (SP) promotes growth, unburdens (S) helps live up to expectations, has a calming and motivating effect (M) helps remain focused under intensive strain (B) helps with problems of the stomach, intestine, discs, joints and meniscus (knee).
Bib.: 2 | 4 | 5 | 8 | 9 | 11 | 17   **Rarity:** readily available ∅

Astrophyllite in Syenite

Mineralogy: astrophyllite: alkaline group silicate (tric., prim.)
Indications: (SP) inspiration, truthfulness (S) receptive to needs, lively dreams (M) helps catch up on unfinished projects, openness, expressive ability (B) for the large intestine and hormone system, very helpful with menstrual and menopausal problems.
Bib.: 2 | 4 | 6 | 8   **Rarity:** scarce ∅

Augite

Mineralogy: chain silicate of the pyroxene group (mon., prim./tert.)
Indications: (SP) composure, stability (S) relieves pressure and strain; gives self-assurance (M) supports active defence against oppressive influences (B) helps with problems of the digestive system and the back, especially those caused by emotional strain.
Bib.: 2 | 4 | 6 | 8   **Rarity:** not always available ○

Auripigmentum (Orpiment)

Mineralogy: yellow arsenic sulphide (mon., prim.)
Indications: (SP) brings intensity to life, vitality (S) peps up, stimulates enjoyment of life, increases sexual desire (M) makes alert and enhances quick intellectual grasp (B) promotes a turnaround in cases of chronic weakness and debilitating illnesses.
Bib.: 4 | 6   **Rarity:** rare ○

Aurora Quartz (Quartz)

Mineralogy: clear quartz with iridescent zones (trig., sec.)
Indications: (SP) cohesion, unity (S) helps with loneliness, grief and the feeling of not being understood (M) enables perception of all aspects of life (B) frees breathing, helps with constrictions, good for the lungs, respiratory tract, eyes and ears.
Bib.: 4   **Rarity:** rare ○

Aventurine Quartz, blue (Dumortierite Quartzite)
Mineralogy: glittering quartz containing dumortierite (rhom./trig., tert.)
Indications: **(SP)** imperturbability **(S)** calms, relaxes, relieves nervousness **(M)** helps approach interesting or important projects calmly but with determination **(B)** ameliorates pain and chronic stiffness; has a cooling effect and reduces fever.
Bib.: 4–6 | 8 | 19   Rarity: scarce ○

Aventurine Quartz, green (Fuchsite Quartzite)
Mineralogy: glittering quartz containing fuchsite (mon./trig., tert.)
Indications: **(SP)** easy-goingness **(S)** helps with nervousness, stress and sleep disorders **(M)** helps free from anxiety and roving thoughts **(B)** protects against heart attack and arteriosclerosis; alleviates rashes, inflammations, sunburn and sunstroke.
Bib.: 1 – 14 | 17–19   Rarity: common ○

Aventurine Quartz, orange (Hematite Quartzite)
Mineralogy: glittering quartz containing hematite (trig., tert.)
Indications: **(SP)** cheerfulness **(S)** promotes a cheerful and relaxed atmosphere **(M)** enables living one's dreams, promotes a relaxed alertness **(B)** promotes blood formation, good blood circulation, warms up and revitalises numb parts of the body, fortifies the liver and senses.
Bib.: 4 | 5 | 6 | 8 | 19   Rarity: rare ◯

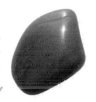

Aventurine Quartz, red (Hematite Quartzite)
Mineralogy: glittering quartz containing hematite (trig., tert.)
Indications: **(SP)** level-headedness **(S)** conveys strength and self-assurance **(M)** helps pursue personal goals in a pragmatic manner **(B)** stimulates blood circulation, enhances blood flow, nerves and perceptive abilities of the senses and enhances muscle strength.
Bib.: 4–6 | 8 | 19   Rarity: rare ◯

Aventurine Quartz, red (Piemontite Quartzite)
Mineralogy: glittering quartz containing piemontite (mon./trig., tert.)
Indications: **(SP)** generosity, enjoyment **(S)** makes hearty, hopeful, courageous and helps express needs **(M)** makes understanding, curious and thirsty for knowledge **(B)** promotes virility and strengthens the genitals, kidneys, liver, small intestines, heart and nerves.
Bib.: 4–6 | 8   Rarity: not always available ◯

Aventurine Quartz, white (Muscovite Quartzite)

Mineralogy: glittering quartz containing muscovite (mon./trig., tert.)
Indications: (SP) common sense, honesty (S) helps conduct oneself with comportment and self-confidence (M) makes cautious, helps reflect carefully and make intelligent decisions (B) helps with nervousness, trembling, unwell feeling and breaking into a sweat.
Bib.: 4–6 | 8   **Rarity:** rare ○

Axinite

Mineralogy: calcium aluminium boron silicate (tric., tert.)
Indications: (SP) for determination (S) helps pluck up courage and strengthen hope and trust (M) lends to right insight when in doubt (B) helps with sensory and motor disorders, paralysis, neuropathies, migraine and vegetative dystonia.
Bib.: 4 | 6 | 8   **Rarity:** scarce ○

Azurite

Mineralogy: alkaline copper carbonate (mon., prim./sec.)
Indications: (SP) recognition, experience (S) reveals and helps give up adopted unexamined ideas (M) makes reflective, critical, enhances awareness and self-recognition (B) stimulates the liver, brain, nerves and thyroid gland; improves reflex actions.
Bib.: 1 | 2 | 4–6 | 8 | 14 | 19   **Rarity:** readily available ⊘

Azurite-Malachite

Mineralogy: alkaline copper carbonate (mon., prim./sec.)
Indications: (SP) harmony, interest (S) makes open-minded, helpful and disperses inner turmoil (M) harmonises the intellect and feelings, helps resolve conflicts (B) normalises disharmonious cell growth, releases cramps, fortifies the liver and detoxifies.
Bib.: 1 | 2 | 4 | 6–8 | 19   **Rarity:** scarce ⊘

Barite, brown (Heavy Spar)

Mineralogy: brown barium sulphate (rhom., prim./sec./tert.)
Indications: (SP) stability, self-assurance (S) increases performance and promotes independence (M) helps to substantiate ideas and visions (B) improves posture, helps with weariness, sore throat and stomach ache and reduces the effects of radiation.
Bib.: 2 | 4 | 6 | 8 | 9   **Rarity:** not always available ○

Barite, red (Heavy Spar)

Mineralogy: red barium sulphate (rhom., prim.)

Indications: (SP) standpoint, self-assertion (S) helps with feeling of despondency and inferiority (M) enables prolonged concentration during mental fatigue (B) helps with muscle weakness, strong sensitivity to cold, and reduces the effects of radiation.

Bib.: 2 | 4 | 6 | 8 | 9   **Rarity:** not always available ⌀

Barite, white (Heavy Spar)

Mineralogy: white barium sulphate (rhom., prim./sec./tert.)

Indications: (SP) setting boundaries, importance (S) clears confusion, helps with shyness and anxiety (M) strengthens memory, helps formulate thoughts and words (B) helps with diseases of the skin and glands, swollen lymph nodes and effects of radiation.

Bib.: 2 | 4 | 6 | 8 | 9   **Rarity:** not always available ○

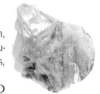

Basalt

Mineralogy: volcanic rock with low silica content (mon./tric., prim.)

Indications: (SP) well rooted (S) strengthens the inner connection to oneself and others (M) urges one to act according to one's inner truth (B) alleviates chronic tension, headache, migraine, back pain, pains and constipation.

Bib.: 2 | 4 | 6 | 8   **Rarity:** readily available ⌀

Beryl, colourless (Goshenite)

Mineralogy: beryllium aluminium ring silicate (hex., prim.)

Indications: (SP) goal-oriented, efficient (S) promotes patience, perseverance, discipline and open-heartedness (M) aids intensive learning, care and systematic approach (B) helps with short- and long-sightedness; strengthens the nerves, relieves nausea and pain.

Bib.: 1 | 2 | 4 | 6 | 8 | 16   **Rarity:** rare ⌀

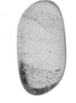

Beryl, red (Bixbite)

Mineralogy: beryl containing manganese and lithium (hexag., prim.)

Indications: (SP) energises and makes dynamic (S) helps with lack of drive, over-exertion and disharmony (M) lends vigour to tackle long-postponed unpleasant or difficult issues (B) fortifies circulatory system and nerves; helps with the results of permanent stress.

Bib.: 1 | 2 | 4 | 6 | 8 | 19   **Rarity:** rare ⌀

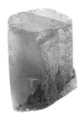

Beryl (Vanadium Beryl)

Mineralogy: beryl containing vanadium (hex., prim.)
Indications: (SP) care, trust (S) helps with lack of courage and despair (M) motivates to tackle the seemingly impossible (B) fortifies the liver and functional tissue of the organs (parenchyma); detoxifies; helps with inflammations and degeneration processes.
Bib.: 2 | 4 | 6 | 8   **Rarity:** scarce

Biotite Lenses (Birthing Stones)

Mineralogy: magnesium iron mica (mon., tert.)
Indications: (SP) aids self-realisation (S) protects from external influences (M) helps with decision-making (B) helps with hyperacidity, rheumatism, gout, constipation, sciatica and kidney problems; aids childbirth (triggers labour, relaxes the pelvis and softens the neck of the womb).
Bib.: 1–6 | 8 | 9   **Rarity:** rare

Blue Quartz (Dumortierite Quartzite)

Mineralogy: quartz with dumortierite inclusions (trig./rhom., tert.)
Indications: (SP) lightness (S) helps with anger, commotion, stress, eases mood swings and brings emotional calm (M) boosts learning through listening and empathising (B) relieves stress-induced skin reactions, calms the nerves and pulse, cools and relaxes.
Bib.: 4 | 6 | 8 | 19   **Rarity:** not always available

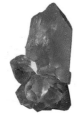

Blue Quartz (Indigolite Quartz, Olenite Quartz)

Mineralogy: quartz with tourmaline inclusions (trig., prim.)
Indications: (SP) sense of reality (S) brings the feeling of expanse and lightness, enhances sexual control especially during premature ejaculation (M) promotes pragmatic thinking and action (B) eases pain, has a cooling and fever-reducing effect, helps with bronchitis.
Bib.: 2 | 4 | 6 | 19   **Rarity:** rare

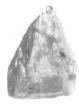

Brasilianite

Mineralogy: anhydrous, alkaline phosphate (mon., prim.)
Indications: (SP) guidance by the higher self (S) helps with nightmares, fear and insomnia (M) aids viewing things from a higher standpoint (B) ameliorates recurring pain, including menstrual pain.
Bib.: 2 | 4 | 6 | 8   **Rarity:** scarce

Bronzite (Ferro-Enstatite)

Mineralogy: chain silicate of the pyroxene group (rhom., prim./tert.)
Indications: (SP) for inner composure (S) lends vigour and inner calm simultaneously, as well as regeneration from chronic exhaustion (M) helps retain a clear head and control under permanent stress (B) fortifies the nerves, releases cramps and relieves pain.
Bib.: 2–6 | 8 | 14   **Rarity:** readily available ○

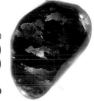

Bronzite Gabbro (Gabbro)

Mineralogy: gabbro with bronzite and labradorite (rhom./tric., prim.)
Indications: (SP) observance, holistic comprehension (S) strengthens and fortifies, promotes attentiveness (M) brings deep understanding through intensive examination (B) fortifies the kidneys, helps with ear diseases and promotes sense of hearing.
Bib.: 4   **Rarity:** scarce ○

Bronzite Peridotite

Mineralogy: meta-peridotite containing bronzite (rhom., tert.)
Indications: (SP) dedication, steadfastness (S) enables conserving one's energy and not exhausting oneself (M) helps care for oneself and put a limit on demands made by others (B) eases cramps and pains, helps with rheumatism and gout.
Bib.: 4   **Rarity:** rare ⊘

Budstone (Greenschist)

Mineralogy: rock with feldspar and fuchsite (tric./mon., tert.)
Indications: (SP) self-control (S) makes it easier to let go rage and fury (M) helps to retain self-control under emotional onslaughts (B) alleviates effects of radiation, sunburn, sunstroke, heatstroke and insect bites; helps with problems of the bladder.
Bib.: 1–6 | 8 | 9 | 13 | 14 | 16 | 17   **Rarity:** not always available ○

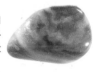

Bustamite

Mineralogy: wollastonite containing manganese (tric., tert.)
Indications: (SP) deepens connection with the earth, inner composure (S) promotes ability to relax, lends positive disposition to physical nature (M) helps focus thoughts and turn them into deeds (B) enhances motor nerves as well as sensation in legs and feet.
Bib.: 2 | 4 | 6 | 8   **Rarity:** scarce ○

Calcite, blue
Mineralogy: blue calcium carbonate (trig., sec.)
Indications: **(SP)** sense of judgement **(S)** calms, makes inwardly stable and confident in appearance **(M)** improves memory and powers of discernment **(B)** good for the lymph, mucous membranes, skin, large intestine, connective tissues, bones and teeth.
Bib.: 1–9 | 13 | 14 | 17 | 19   **Rarity:** readily available

Calcite, green
Mineralogy: green calcium carbonate (trig., sec.)
Indications: **(SP)** makes imaginative **(S)** aids letting go of constraining emotions **(M)** makes more open and interested, helps transform ideas into action **(B)** alleviates inflammation; enhances detoxification; helps with problems of the liver and gallbladder.
Bib.: 1–8 | 13 | 14 | 16 | 17 | 19   **Rarity:** common

Calcite, honey-coloured 'Honey Calcite'
Mineralogy: iron-containing calcium carbonate (trig., sec.)
Indications: **(SP)** assurance **(S)** promotes a confident and optimistic approach to life **(M)** initiates relying more on one's feeling and sensing **(B)** stimulates digestion, metabolism and excretion; strengthens the intestine, connective tissues, bones and teeth.
Bib.: 1–8 | 13 | 14 | 16 | 17 | 19   **Rarity:** readily available

Calcite 'Iceland Spar'
Mineralogy: clear calcite with rhombohedral termination (trig., sec.)
Indications: **(SP)** presence of mind **(S)** helps overcome laziness and free oneself from guilty conscience **(M)** enables drawing unprejudiced, clear conclusions **(B)** cleanses the intestines, improves excretion and helps with calcium deficiency.
Bib.: 2 | 4–6 | 8   **Rarity:** not always available

Calcite, orange 'Orange Calcite'
Mineralogy: iron-containing calcium carbonate (trig., sec.)
Indications: **(SP)** self-confidence **(S)** promotes self-respect and confidence in one's abilities **(M)** promotes optimism, without becoming unrealistic **(B)** enhances digestion and healing of the connective tissues, skin and bones.
Bib.: 1–14 | 16 | 17 | 18 | 19   **Rarity:** common

Calcite, pink 'Mangano Calcite'

Mineralogy: manganese-containing calcium carbonate (trig., sec.)
Indications: (SP) friendliness **(S)** promotes warmth, acceptance, helpfulness, friendly disposition **(M)** makes open-minded and accommodating of others **(B)** strengthens the heart, normalises heartbeat; good for connective tissues, blood vessels and skin.
Bib.: 1–9 | 11 | 13 | 14   **Rarity:** readily available

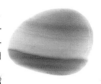

Calcite, red

Mineralogy: iron-containing calcium carbonate (trig., sec.)
Indications: (SP) for willpower **(S)** helps overcome laziness and listlessness **(M)** initiates competent and successful materialisation of ideas **(B)** promotes growth, fortifies immune system, stimulates blood clotting and wound healing and improves quality of the blood.
Bib.: 1–9 | 13 | 14 | 16 | 19   **Rarity:** readily available

Calcite, white

Mineralogy: calcium carbonate (trig., sec.)
Indications: (SP) for development **(S)** promotes spiritual progress **(M)** makes confident and faster in thinking and acting **(B)** stimulates metabolism; promotes growth in children; fortifies mucous membranes, skin, intestine, connective tissues, bones and teeth.
Bib.: 1–14 | 16–18 | 19   **Rarity:** common ○

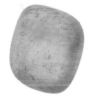

Calcite, yellow, 'Lemon Calcite'

Mineralogy: iron-containing calcium carbonate (trig., sec.)
Indications: (SP) self-esteem **(S)** fortifies sense of security, self-esteem and joie de vivre **(M)** makes resolute in disputes **(B)** stimulates food digestion, assimilation and metabolism; strengthens the skin, connective tissues, bones and teeth.
Bib.: 1–7 | 11 | 13 | 14 | 16 | 19   **Rarity:** common

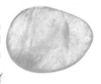

Carnelian, banded, 'Carnelian Agate' (Chalcedony)

Mineralogy: carnelian coloured agate (quartz, trig., prim./sec.)
Indications: (SP) stimulates, motivates **(S)** helps overcome difficulties and energetically defend a cause **(M)** enhances receptivity **(B)** stimulates assimilation of vitamins, nutrients and minerals in the small intestine; improves blood viscosity.
Bib.: 1–9 | 11–14 | 16 | 19   **Rarity:** not always available

Carnelian (Chalcedony)

Mineralogy: chalcedony containing hematite (quartz, trig., prim./sec.)
Indications: (SP) courage, willpower (S) promotes vigour, courage, stability and good moods (M) promotes idealism, sense of community and pragmatism (B) improves quality of the blood; stimulates the small intestine, metabolism, circulation, blood flow.
Bib.: 1–9 | 11–14 | 16 | 19   Rarity: not always available

Cassiterite

Mineralogy: tin oxide (rutile group, tetr., prim./tert.)
Indications: (SP) greatness, perfection (S) promotes generosity in the right measure (M) helps realise dreams and perceive many things objectively (B) helps with eating disorders, emaciation or excess weight; has a regulating effect on the nerves and hormone system.
Bib.: 2 | 4 | 6 | 8   Rarity: scarce ○

Cat's Eye Quartz (Aqualite, Schiller Quartz) (Quartz)

Mineralogy: quartz with hornblende fibre (trig./mon., tert.)
Indications: (SP) insight, detachment (S) aids setting boundaries and helps overcome great barriers at the same time (M) makes it easier to grasp complex contexts (B) relieves pain; calms the nerves; helps with hormonal hyperactivity.
Bib.: 2 | 8   Rarity: not always available ○

Cavansite

Mineralogy: calcium vanadium sheet silicate (rhom., sec.)
Indications: (SP) self-respect, sense of beauty (S) for encouragement and optimism, makes life-affirming (M) inspiration, learning ability, logical thinking (B) for cleansing and regeneration; helps with problems of the kidneys, bladder and ears (tinnitus).
Bib.: 2 | 4 | 6 | 8 | 9   Rarity: scarce

Chalcedony, blue

Mineralogy: fibrous quartz (trig., prim./sec.)
Indications: (SP) presence of mind (S) helps accept new situations and overcome resistance (M) bestows inner calm and relaxed attention (B) stimulates milk production in nursing mothers; helps with sensitivity to weather changes; alleviates diabetes.
Bib.: 1–6 | 8 | 11 | 13 | 14 | 17 | 19   Rarity: readily available ○

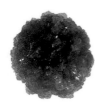

Chalcedony, blue banded, 'Chalcedony Agate'

Mineralogy: fibrous quartz (silicon dioxide, trig., prim.)
Indications: (SP) communication (S) enhances rhetoric and self-expression (M) aids listening, understanding and confiding (B) promotes flow of lymph; helps thyroid gland, kidneys and bladder; helps with hoarseness, colds and allergies, reduces blood pressure and fever.
Bib.: 1–14 | 16 | 17 | 19   **Rarity:** common

Chalcedony 'Chrome Chalcedony'

Mineralogy: chalcedony containing chromium (trig., prim./sec.)
Indications: (SP) carefree (S) bestows a light-hearted disposition to life; helps face up to worries and unpleasant matters (M) helps remain open to new ideas (B) has an anti-inflammatory effect, also on rheumatic diseases, polyarthritis among others
Bib.: 1 | 2 | 4–6 | 8   **Rarity:** not always available

Chalcedony 'Copper Chalcedony'

Mineralogy: copper-containing chalcedony (trig., sec.)
Indications: (SP) for enjoyment, harmony (S) aids sensuality, openness and friendliness (M) promotes sense of judgement, tolerance, objective approach and sense of beauty (B) detoxifies; inhibits inflammations; helps with fungal infections; fortifies the immune system.
Bib.: 1 | 2 | 4–6 | 8   **Rarity:** scarce

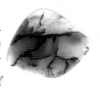

Chalcedony 'Dendritic Chalcedony'

Mineralogy: chalcedony with manganese dendrites (trig., prim./sec.)
Indications: (SP) breaks habits (S) frees from unconscious mechanisms, habits and moods (M) aids precise thinking and attentive listening (B) activates cleansing of the lymph system, mucous membranes and respiratory tract; eases after-effects of smoking.
Bib.: 1 | 2 | 4–6 | 8   **Rarity:** readily available

Chalcedony, green

Mineralogy: chalcedony with iron silicates (quartz, trig., prim.)
Indications: (SP) forbearance, consideration (S) promotes a considerate attitude towards oneself and others (M) helps expend one's energy rationally (B) fortifies the immune reaction; improves well-being; helps with infections and enhances the senses.
Bib.: 1 | 2 | 4–6 | 8   **Rarity:** not always available

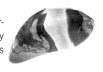

Chalcedony, pink 'Rose Chalcedony'
Mineralogy: chalcedony containing manganese (trig., prim./sec.)
Indications: (SP) for warm-heartedness **(S)** makes lively, kind and helpful **(M)** promotes openness and understanding **(B)** stimulates milk production in nursing mothers; helps with diabetes, colds and heart diseases caused by protracted infections.
Bib.: 1–6 | 8 | 9 | 11 | 14 | 17   **Rarity:** readily available ○

Chalcedony, red 'Blood Chalcedony'
Mineralogy: iron-containing chalcedony (trig., prim./sec.)
Indications: (SP) vigour, flexibility **(S)** enhances strength, vitality and vigour **(M)** fortifies willpower; keeps flexible while retaining one's standpoint **(B)** stabilises blood circulation, stimulates blood clotting and aids wound healing.
Bib.: 1 | 2 | 4–6 | 8 | 9 | 11   **Rarity:** readily available ○

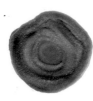

Chalcedony, rosette
Mineralogy: petal-like chalcedony formations (trig., prim.)
Indications: (SP) helps unfold **(S)** makes sociable and receptive **(M)** helps be oneself, express oneself clearly **(B)** helps problems of the stomach, skin, mucous membranes, respiratory tract, glands, tissues and sensory organs (depending on shape of petal-like formation).
Bib.: 1–6 | 8 | 9   **Rarity:** readily available ○

Chalcedony, yellow (Carnelian yellow)
Mineralogy: chalcedony containing limonite (quartz, trig., prim.)
Indications: (SP) for modesty **(S)** makes content with very little, promotes contentment and joy **(M)** brings stability in thoughts and actions; helps find simple solutions **(B)** helps with weak circulation; aids digestion and elimination.
Bib.: 2 | 4–6 | 8 | 19   **Rarity:** readily available ⊘

Chalcopyrite
Mineralogy: copper iron sulphide (tetr., prim./sec./tert.)
Indications: (SP) curiosity, experience **(S)** exposes hidden causes of problems and illnesses **(M)** promotes the desire to understand life, improves power of observation and systematic thinking **(B)** promotes cleansing and excretion (intestine).
Bib.: 2 | 4–6 | 8   **Rarity:** readily available ⊘

Chalcopyrite Nephrite

Mineralogy: chalcopyrite nephrite mixture (tetr./mon., tert.)
Indications: (SP) for insight, experience (S) reveals one's less pleasant, dark side; helps accept or change it (M) helps learn from mistakes (B) promotes cleansing/excretion through kidneys and intestines.
Bib.: 2 | 4 | 5   Rarity: scarce ○

Charoite

Mineralogy: sheet silicate rich in minerals (mon., tert.)
Indications: (SP) for vigour, determination (S) relaxes, helps overcome obsessions and obstacles (M) helps make important decisions and tackle huge piles of work (B) soothes the nerves, relieves pain and releases cramps.
Bib.: 1 | 2 | 4–9 | 11 | 12 | 14 | 19   Rarity: not always available ⌀

Chert, brown

Mineralogy: jasper opal mixture (trig./am., sec.)
Indications: (SP) productivity (S) reduces stress, relaxes, brings gentle surge of energy (M) helps realise plans in a simple way (B) purifies connective tissues and skin; alleviates allergies; improves intestinal flora and helps with constipation and diarrhoea.
Bib.: 2 | 4 | 6 | 8   Rarity: readily available ⌀

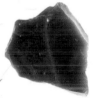

Chert, coloured (Flint coloured)

Mineralogy: jasper opal mixture (trig./am., sec.)
Indications: (SP) exchange, open-mindedness (S) flexibility and composure (M) promotes team spirit (B) purifies connective tissues and skin; good against corns and ganglions; enhances stability of the vessels, digestion and elimination.
Bib.: 2 | 4 | 6 | 8   Rarity: not always available ⌀

Chiastolite (Andalusite)

Mineralogy: aluminium island silicate with carbon (rhom., tert.)
Indications: (SP) identity, helps achieve one's vocation in life (S) helps overcome fear and feeling of guilt (M) promotes sense of reality and sobriety (B) alleviates hyperacidity, rheumatism and gout; helps with exhaustion, weakness and symptoms of paralysis.
Bib.: 1 | 2 | 4–6 | 8 | 9 | 14   Rarity: scarce ⌀

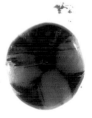

Chrome Diopside

Mineralogy: diopside containing chrome (chain silicate, mon., tert.)
Indications: (SP) mental faculty, inspiration (S) helps face life in a carefree manner, makes lively and brings harmony and joie de vivre (M) promotes power of imagination and creativity (B) strengthens the kidneys, senses and nerves; ameliorates local inflammation.
Bib.: 2 | 4–6 | 8   Rarity: scarce

Chrome Grossular (Garnet)

Mineralogy: grossular containing chrome (island silicate, cub., tert.)
Indications: (SP) restorative; aids self-determination (S) brings new drive in times of stagnation (M) revives imagination and creativity (B) fortifies the liver and kidneys; detoxifies and alleviates inflammations; regulates fat metabolism, prevents arteriosclerosis.
Bib.: 2 | 4–6 | 8 | 14   Rarity: scarce

Chrysanthemum Stone (Celestine in Limestone)

Mineralogy: celestine (rhom.) in limestone (trig., sec.)
Indications: (SP) circumspection (S) emotionally stabilizing effect, centring for a positive, solid lifestyle (M) calming, considered, deliberate and slow (B) encourages development of bone and tissue, calms nervous disturbances of internal organs.
Bib.: 4 | 6   Rarity: not always available ○

Chrysoberyl

Mineralogy: aluminium beryllium oxide (rhom., prim./tert.)
Indications: (SP) self-control, discipline (S) helps with fear, feeling of unease, stress, nervousness, hyperactivity (M) promotes concentration, learning ability and strategic thinking (B) helps with nerve problems, speech disorders, stammering, sensory disorders; enhances the liver.
Bib.: 1–9 | 12 | 14 | 19   Rarity: scarce ○

Chrysoberyl, Cat's Eye

Mineralogy: chrysoberyl with cat's eye (rhom., prim./tert.)
Indications: (SP) self-determination, conviction (S) aids security, self-confidence and authority (M) helps stand firmly for one's conviction and convince others (B) strengthens the liver, brain, nerves, senses and immune system.
Bib.: 1–7 | 12 | 14 | 19   Rarity: scarce

Chrysocolla
Mineralogy: hydrous copper ring silicate (mon., prim./sec.)
Indications: (SP) balance (S) helps with stress and mood swings (M) helps keep one's cool (B) strengthens the liver; relaxes; helps with infections, sore throat, burns, scars, fever, cramps and menstrual pains.
Bib.: 1–9 | 11–14 | 17 | 19   **Rarity:** readily available ∅

Chrysoprase (Chalcedony)
Mineralogy: chalcedony containing nickel (quartz, trig., sec.)
Indications: (SP) detoxification (S) promotes trust, and sense of safety; helps with heartache, jealousy and nightmares (M) helps solve relationship problems (B) purifies, detoxifies, and helps with allergies, epilepsy, skin diseases, fungal infections and rheumatism.
Bib.: 1–9 | 11–14 | 16 | 17 | 19   **Rarity:** readily available ∅

Celestine
Mineralogy: strontium sulphate (rhom., sec.)
Indications: (SP) relief and stability (S) helps with severe feelings of constriction and unease and fainting fits (M) brings structure into one's life, thoughts and work (B) releases chronic tension and hardenings in bones, tissues and organs.
Bib.: 2 | 4–6 | 8 | 9 | 14   **Rarity:** readily available ∅

Cinnabarite (Cinnabar)
Mineralogy: mercury sulphide (trig., prim./sec.)
Indications: (SP) uncompromising (S) helps with instability, restlessness and nervousness (M) eases concentration problems (B) helps with indurate glands and diseases of the intestine, skin and mucous membranes. **Caution:** may contain metallic mercury – poisonous!
Bib.: 2 | 4–6 | 8   **Rarity:** scarce ○

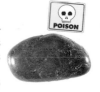

Cinnabarite Opal (Cinnabar Opal)
Mineralogy: opal with cinnabar inclusions (am./trig., prim.)
Indications: (SP) deep cleansing (S) helps transform stubborn destructive patterns (M) makes flexible, capable of learning (B) detoxifies intensively right down to elimination of heavy metals, often with strong initial reactions; helps with tonsillitis and inflammation.
Bib.: 4–6 | 8   **Rarity:** rare ∅

Citrine (Quartz, iron-free)
Mineralogy: yellow crystal quartz (silicon dioxide, trig., prim.)
Indications: (SP) self-assurance (S) makes extrovert and promotes the desire for new experiences (M) helps deal with and understand absorbed impressions (B) fortifies the nerves; helps with sensitivity to weather changes; also helps with bedwetting.
Bib.: 1–9 | 11–14 | 19 | 21   **Rarity:** not always available ◯

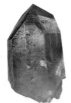

Citrine (Quartz, containing iron)
Mineralogy: crystal quartz containing iron (trig., prim./sec./tert.)
Indications: (SP) gives courage to face life (S) gives joie de vivre; aids self-expression; helps with depression (M) promotes determination and ability to deal with confrontation (B) fortifies the stomach, spleen and pancreas, has a warming effect and enhances performance.
Bib.: 1–9 | 11–14 | 19 | 21   **Rarity:** not always available ⌀

Clear Quartz (Quartz)
Mineralogy: clear crystal quartz (trig., prim./sec./tert.)
Indications: (SP) clarity, neutrality (S) strengthens personal point of view, improves memory (M) improves perceptive faculty, increases awareness and brings clarity in thinking (B) enhances energy flow; fortifies nerves, brain, glands; alleviates pain and swellings.
Bib.: 1–14 | 16–19 | 21   **Rarity:** common ⌀

Clear Quartz 'Accumulation Crystal' (Quartz)
Mineralogy: crystal with edge-like termination (trig., prim./sec./tert.)
Indications: (SP) inner composure (S) has a fortifying effect, helps concentrate energy and manage one's energy (M) promotes calm, level-headed attention (B) helps eliminate excess energy and reduce fever; clears the atmosphere in a room.
Bib.: 2 | 4–6 | 8   **Rarity:** common ⌀

Clear Quartz 'Bridge Crystal' (Quartz)
Mineralogy: small crystal partially covered by a larger one (trig., prim./tert.)
Indications: (SP) unification, understanding (S) reminds of forgotten and neglected needs (M) helps harmonise desires and obligations as well as to reach out to others (B) improves the perception of the body and helps with chronic illnesses.
Bib.: 4 | 21   **Rarity:** scarce ⌀

Clear Quartz 'Cathedral Crystal' (Quartz)

Mineralogy: Crystals formed in the shape of a cathedral (trig., prim./tert.)
Indications: **(SP)** spiritual might **(S)** enhances contemplation and self-awareness **(M)** facilitates drawing from the wealth of knowledge and experience and implementing many ideas **(B)** strengthens the spleen and promotes the vitality of all organs and body functions.
Bib.: 4 | 21   Rarity: scarce ♂

Clear Quartz 'Channelling Crystal' (Quartz)

Min.: quartz crystal w. large 7-sided facet at apex (trig., prim./sec./tert.)
Indications: **(SP)** for receptivity **(S)** enhances intuition, sensitivity and mediumistic abilities, promotes inner calm and open-mindedness **(M)** sharpens receptive faculty, aids meditation **(B)** improves care of one's body and its needs.
Bib.: 2 | 4–6 | 8 | 21   Rarity: not always available ∅

Clear Quartz 'Crystal Cluster' (Quartz)

Min.: crystal with a cluster of smaller crystals (trig., prim./sec./tert.)
Indications: **(SP)** goodwill, responsibility **(S)** helps transform weaknesses into strengths and delve into new experiences **(M)** enhances sharing one's ability and supporting others **(B)** strengthens the nerves, muscles, tendons, joints and limbs.
Bib.: 4 | 6 | 8 | 21   Rarity: not always available ∅

Clear Quartz 'Double Termination' (Quartz)

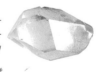

Min.: quartz crystal pointed at both ends (trig., prim./sec./tert.)
Indications: **(SP)** unifies **(S)** improves contact with other beings, enhances memory and dream recall **(M)** promotes understanding, telepathy and helps express oneself clearly **(B)** improves simultaneous flow of energy in two directions and releases blockages.
Bib.: 2–6 | 8 | 18 | 21   Rarity: readily available ∅

Clear Quartz 'Dow Crystal' (Quartz)

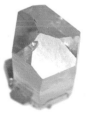

Min.: quartz crystal w. alternate 3- and 7-sided facets (trig., prim./tert.)
Indications: **(SP)** spiritual abilities **(S)** promotes self-harmony **(M)** helps consciously develop and train personal spiritual abilities **(B)** balances energy shortages and excesses in the body organism and promotes its self-organisation.
Bib.: 2 | 4–6 | 8 | 21   Rarity: scarce ∅

Clear Quartz 'Etched Crystal' (Quartz)

Mineralogy: crystal with deep notches (trig., prim./tert.)
Indications: (SP) maturity, experience **(S)** helps deal with experiences and to recall primeval knowledge **(M)** enables a holistic view of things from different perspectives **(B)** enhances rhythmic body processes and accelerates healing processes.
Bib.: 4 | 21   **Rarity:** rare

Clear Quartz 'Faden Quartz' (Quartz)

Mineralogy: crystal cluster with 'growth threads' (trig., tert.)
Indications: (SP) healing **(S)** helps with intense inner conflict and in dealing with painful experiences **(M)** helps unify incompatible circumstances and forges links between people **(B)** alleviates back pain and enormously strengthens self-healing power.
Bib.: 4–6 | 8   **Rarity:** scarce

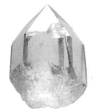

Clear Quartz 'Generator Crystal' (Quartz)

Min.: crystal with 6 equal facets at the peak (trig., prim./sec./tert.)
Indications: (SP) strengthens **(S)** promotes poise, confidence, uprightness **(M)** aids in concise expression of thoughts and words **(B)** directs energy flow to the extremities and fortifies and stimulates the meridians and nerves.
Bib.: 2 | 4–6 | 8 | 21   **Rarity:** scarce

Clear Quartz 'Harmony Quartz', 'Self-Healer' (Quartz)

Mineralogy: self-healed crystal (trig., prim./sec./tert.)
Indications: (SP) amendment **(S)** helps come to terms with blows of fate and resolve conflicts in relationships **(M)** makes it possible to draw positive lessons even from painful experiences **(B)** stimulates self-healing power; helps with infections and fractures.
Bib.: 2 | 4 | 6 | 8 | 21   **Rarity:** not always available

Clear Quartz 'Herkimer Quartz' (Quartz)

Mineralogy: double-terminated crystal from Herkimer/USA (trig., sec.)
Indications: (SP) awareness, clarity **(S)** improves dream recall and emotional orientation **(M)** enhances awareness and heightens consciousness **(B)** relieves pain (by placing three crystals in a triangle); supports the nerves, brain and senses.
Bib.: 2–6 | 8 | 18   **Rarity:** rare

Clear Quartz 'Isis Crystal' (Quartz)

Min.: crystal with a 5-sided face (trig., prim./tert.)
Indications: (SP) further development (S) helps overcome loss, suffering and injustice (M) promotes honesty and uprightness, helps correct mistakes and reorientate oneself (B) enhances regeneration, self-healing energies and the immune system.
Bib.: 4 | 21   **Rarity:** scarce

Clear Quartz 'Laser Quartz' (Quartz)

Mineralogy: crystal w. steep rhombohedron surfaces (trig., prim./tert.)
Indications: (SP) promotes focus (S) helps concentrate one's energy and mobilise reserves (M) strengthens mental intention, focuses thoughts on current goal (B) directs energy flow towards the apex; has a strong stimulating effect on the meridians and nerves.
Bib.: 2 | 4–6 | 8 | 13 | 14 | 21   **Rarity:** not always available

Clear Quartz 'Lightning Strike Quartz' (Quartz)

Mineralogy: crystal with lightning-strike indentations (trig., tert.)
Indications: (SP) heightens consciousness (S) strengthens the intuition and intensifies dream experience (M) promotes consciousness, alertness, ability to deal with confrontation and flashes of inspiration (B) gives energy, intensifies cleansing and excretion, regulates menstruation.
Bib.: 4 | 6   **Rarity:** rare

Clear Quartz 'Manifestation Crystal' (Quartz)

Min.: small crystal enclosed within a larger crystal (trig., prim./tert.)
Indications: (SP) prosperity, blossoming (S) nourishes and gives space to our inner requests (M) stimulates transforming one's plans and decisions into deeds (B) strengthens the backbone and muscles, boosts the stomach, spleen, liver, gallbladder, kidneys and bladder.
Bib.: 4 | 21   **Rarity:** rare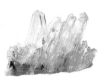

Clear Quartz 'Needle Quartz' (Quartz)

Mineralogy: needle-like long prismatic crystals (trig., tert.)
Indications: (SP) flow, alignment (S) sets internal images, recollections and feelings into motion (M) motivates to spiritual advancement and success (B) fortifies the nerves, regulates and controls energy flow in the body, helps harmonise scars.
Bib.: 2 | 4–6 | 8   **Rarity:** scarce ○

Clear Quartz 'Phantom Quartz' (Quartz)

Min.: quartz crystal with visible young forms (trig., prim./sec./tert.)
Indications: (SP) overcoming boundaries **(S)** helps overcome fear, makes courageous (and confident in one's abilities) **(M)** helps to extend the boundaries of one's thoughts and to think and do the 'impossible' **(B)** enhances growth and development of the body.
Bib.: 1 | 2 | 4–6 | 8 | 21   Rarity: scarce

Clear Quartz 'Phantom Quartz' with Chlorite (Quartz)

Mineralogy: crystal with with chlorite phantom (trig., tert.)
Indications: (SP) growth, stages of development **(S)** gives faith and courage to face life **(M)** opens up unexpected new horizons and helps awaken unknown abilities **(B)** stimulates growth in children; aids regeneration and fortifies the immune system.
Bib.: 2 | 4–6 | 8   Rarity: scarce

Clear Quartz 'Rainbow Crystal' (Quartz)

Min.: crystal with colourful light reflection (trig., prim./sec./tert.)
Indications: (SP) fascination **(S)** alleviates worries and sorrow, brings joy and encourages one to participate in the colourful game of life **(M)** helps transform negative thoughts and develop interest **(B)** enhances all the senses, eases constrictions and breathing.
Bib.: 4 | 6 | 8 | 19 | 21   Rarity: readily available ○

Clear Quartz 'Receiver Crystal' (Quartz)

Min.: quartz crystal with very large surface tip (trig., prim./tert.)
Indications: (SP) brings relief **(S)** releases tension, has an emotionally refreshing and fortifying effect **(M)** helps redirect fixed attention, allowing better experience of wider environment **(B)** has fever-reducing effect; relaxes; enhances energy flow and detoxification.
Bib.: 2–5 | 8 | 10 | 18   Rarity: readily available

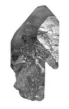

Clear Quartz 'Sceptre Quartz' (Quartz)

Min.: base crystal with new crystal on top (trig., prim./sec./tert.)
Indications: (SP) authority, power **(S)** enables overcoming (recurring) difficulties and to win **(M)** helps recognition of how we shape our reality **(B)** strengthens the brain, nerves, glands, spleen, bladder and genitals.
Bib.: 4 | 6 | 21   Rarity: rare ○

Clear Quartz 'Seed Crystal' (Quartz)

Mineralogy: conically tapering crystal (trig., prim./sec./tert.)
Indications: (SP) initiative, attainment (S) helps start off anew time and again (M) motivates to experiment with different routes to achieve ideas (B) harmonises rhythmic functions like breathing, heartbeat and pulsation of the body fluids.
Bib.: 4 | 21   **Rarity:** scarce ○

Clear Quartz 'Shaman Dow Crystal' (Quartz)

Mineralogy: Dow crystal with phantom (trig., prim./tert.)
Indications: (SP) self-healing (S) provides deep trust in the right and meaningful development of life (M) helps strive for perfection and practise consideration at the same time (B) balances out energy distribution and fortifies self-healing energies.
Bib.: 4 | 21   **Rarity:** rare

Clear Quartz 'Skeleton Quartz', 'Elestial' (Quartz)

Mineralogy: crystal with skeletal growth (trig., sec./tert.)
Indications: (SP) primeval knowledge (S) promotes instinctual trust, increase in strength and swift spontaneous developments (M) helps discover and express one's own primeval knowledge (B) enhances and accelerates development and regeneration processes in the body.
Bib.: 2 | 4–6 | 8   **Rarity:** scarce ⊘

Clear Quartz 'Sprouting Quartz' (Quartz)

Mineralogy: crystal with many small sprouts (trig., prim./sec./tert.)
Indications: (SP) opulence (S) has a building up and reviving effect, makes creative and agile (M) helps mobilising energy to achieve great things with minimal means (B) energises and prevents over-exertion at the same time, strengthens spleen, pancreas and intestines.
Bib.: 4 | 6 | 8   **Rarity:** scarce ◌

Clear Quartz 'Tabular Crystal' (Quartz)

Mineralogy: very wide flat quartz crystal (trig., prim./tert.)
Indications: (SP) broadens horizon (S) promotes sense of community and putting one's own ego last (M) aids circumspection for necessities of overriding importance, helps with ability to prioritise and with mindfulness (B) increases physical energy when necessary.
Bib.: 2 | 4–6 | 8 | 21   **Rarity:** scarce ⊘

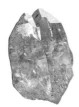

Clear Quartz 'Tantric Twin Crystals' (Quartz)
Mineralogy: formation of conjoined crystals (trig., prim./sec./tert.)
Indications: (SP) relationship, unity **(S)** promotes harmony with one-self and with the environment **(M)** helps accept others, find common interests, communicate frankly and develop understanding **(B)** alleviates allergies and food intolerances.
Bib.: 4 | 21   **Rarity:** not always available

Clear Quartz 'Transmitter Crystal' (Quartz)
Min.: a triangle facet between two 7-sided facets (trig., prim./tert.)
Indications: (SP) links to pure vibrations **(S)** helps alleviate guilty conscience by encouraging confession, heart-to-heart talk and rec-onciliation **(M)** enhances hearing of one's inner voice **(B)** improves communication with the body.
Bib.: 2 | 4–6 | 8 | 21   **Rarity:** scarce

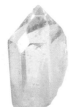

Clear Quartz 'Window Crystal' (Quartz)
Mineralogy: quartz crystal with rhom. facet (trig., prim./tert.)
Indications: (SP) self-recognition, reflection **(S)** brings insight into one's emotional life, promotes untapped abilities **(M)** promotes per-ception and objective self-examination **(B)** helps break resistance against recovery.
Bib.: 2 | 4–6 | 8 | 21   **Rarity:** not always available

Clinoptilolite
Mineralogy: mostly fine-grained zeolite leaves (mon., prim.)
Indications: (SP) cohesion **(S)** enhances a positive attitude to life, reduces stress, brings rejuvenation in sleep **(M)** makes gentle and considerate **(B)** detoxifies, purifies, cleanses the intestine and skin, relieves inflammations, rheumatism, gout, allergies, weak immunity.
Bib.: 2 | 4 | 6   **Rarity:** readily available

Conglomerate 'Goldstone'
Mineralogy: pyrite quartz rock (cub./trig., sec.)
Indications: (SP) self-assessment, self-recognition **(S)** helps confront one's dark side **(M)** improves the assessment of one's energy and abil-ities **(B)** stimulates intensive purification and elimination processes.
Bib.: 2 | 4 | 8   **Rarity:** scarce

Conglomerate 'Brecciated Jasper'
Mineralogy: coarse grainy sediment (mainly trig., sec.)
Indications: (SP) criticism and correction (S) improves one's sense of enhancing or hindering influences (M) triggers continual self-questioning, enabling correction of one's intentions (B) fortifies circulation, the spleen, small intestine and digestion.
Bib.: 2 | 4   **Rarity:** scarce ○

Copal
Mineralogy: dried resin (organic, am., sec.)
Indications: (SP) life-affirming (S) boosts joie de vivre, cheerfulness and resilience (M) brings acceptance, positive thinking, learning ability and willingness to perform (B) loosens mucus, helps with stomach, dental and joint problems, good for the skin, hair and nails.
Bib.: 2 | 4 | 6 | 19   **Rarity:** common ⌀

Copper
Mineralogy: precious metal (natural element, cub., prim./sec.)
Indications: (SP) beauty (S) promotes sense of aesthetics, harmony and love for all beings (M) lends playful creativity and promotes sense of justice (B) for fertility; eases cramps and menstrual pains; fortifies the liver and brain.
Bib.: 2 | 4 | 6 | 8   **Rarity:** readily available ⌀

Cordierite (Iolite, Dichroite)
Min.: aluminium ring silicate with magnesium and iron (rhom., tert.)
Indications: (SP) firmness (S) self-assurance; endurance in adverse situations (M) helps take on responsibility and fulfil duties (B) strengthens the nerves, helps with paralysis and numb limbs, and bearing pain.
Bib.: 2 | 4–6 | 8 | 14   **Rarity:** readily available ○

Cordierite 'Iolite Sunstone', 'Aventurine Cordierite'
Mineralogy: cordierite with hematite inclusions (rhom., tert.)
Indications: (SP) willpower (S) hope in difficult situations (M) aids ability to draw spiritual benefit from defeats (B) releases cramps, boosts performance, stabilises the circulation and helps with fainting fits.
Bib.: 4–6 | 8 | 11   **Rarity:** scarce ○

Covellite
Mineralogy: blue (wet violet) copper sulphide (hex., sec.)
Indications: (SP) self-love, self-recognition (S) helps with discontentment, arrogance and vanity (M) helps accept oneself as one is (B) improves feeling of well-being; harmonises stress and rest; promotes digestion, detoxification and sexuality.
Bib.: 2 | 4 | 6 | 8 | 9   **Rarity:** scarce ⌀

Dalmatian Stone (Aplite)
Mineralogy: granite gangue rock (trig./mon., prim.)
Indications: (SP) reflection (S) has a fortifying, restorative and harmonising effect (M) prompts one to plan carefully, reflect on every phase of development and to carry out plans with vigour (B) stabilises blood circulation, stimulates the nerves and reflex actions.
Bib.: 2 | 4–6 | 8 | 17   **Rarity:** readily available ⌀

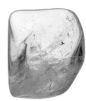

Danburite, colourless
Mineralogy: calcium boron lattice silicate (rhom., prim./sec./tert.)
Indications: (SP) for selflessness, spiritual orientation (S) self-acceptance, unconditional love (M) helps accept people and situations as they are (B) helps with problems of the nerves, brain and digestion with underlying emotional cause.
Bib.: 2 | 4–6 | 8   **Rarity:** not always available ○

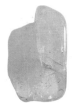

Danburite, pink
Mineralogy: pink calcium boron lattice silicate (rhom., tert.)
Indications: (SP) for charity and humaneness (S) helps overcome possessive and domineering behavioural patterns (M) supports positive thinking (B) helps with problems of the nerves, brain, heart and circulation with underlying emotional cause.
Bib.: 2 | 4 | 5   **Rarity:** scarce ○

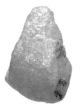

Danburite, yellow
Mineralogy: yellow calcium boron lattice silicate (rhom., tert.)
Indications: (SP) for cheerfulness, assistance (S) promotes self-assurance, helps overcome constraining behavioural patterns (M) improves self-control (B) helps with metabolic disorders and digestion problems with underlying emotional causes, including anorexia.
Bib.: 2 | 4 | 5   **Rarity:** scarce ○

Diamond, black
Mineralogy: black diamond (natural element, cub., tert.)
Indications: (SP) integration (S) helps accept one's dark side and to work on overcoming it (M) helps ward off harmful influences (B) detoxifies, improves excretion, helps with ailments of the bladder and prostate, fortifies the hormonal glands and immune system.
Bib.: 2 | 4–6 | 19   Rarity: readily available

Diamond, colourless
Mineralogy: pure carbon (natural element, cub., tert.)
Indications: (SP) indomitable (S) promotes strength of character, ethics and faithfulness to oneself (M) makes responsible and objective (B) purifies and strengthens the brain, nerves, sensory organs, glands and blood vessels, helps with strokes.
Bib.: 1–9 | 12–14 | 16 | 19   Rarity: readily available

Diamond, grey
Mineralogy: diamond containing boron (natural element, cub., tert.)
Indications: (SP) immortality (S) promotes self-determination and inner stability (M) urges one to do what one recognises to be right and important (B) has a cleansing effect, fortifies the brain, nerves and blood vessels, helps with sense of balance disorders and stroke.
Bib.: 1–9 | 12–14 | 16 | 19   Rarity: readily available

Diamond, yellow
Mineralogy: yellow diamond containing nitrogen (cub., tert.)
Indications: (SP) virtuousness (S) helps remain friendly, just and honest (M) promotes spiritual development and goodwill towards others (B) boosts the spleen, stomach, pancreas and digestion, strengthens the brain, nerves and blood vessels.
Bib.: 1–9 | 12–14 | 16 | 19   Rarity: not always available

Diaspore
Mineralogy: aluminium oxy-hydroxide (rhom., tert.)
Indications: (SP) revives original objectives (S) for perception and change of relationship structures (M) triggers self-analysis and change of one's life (B) promotes digestion, de-acidifies and helps with heartburn and stomach problems.
Bib.: 3 | 4 | 6 | 8 | 9 | 14   Rarity: scarce

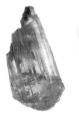

Diopside, black
Mineralogy: pyroxene mineral (chain silicate, mon., prim./ tert.)
Indications: (SP) for forgiveness, letting go (S) helps let go of old pains and wounds (M) helps approach others and make peace (B) boosts the kidneys and harmonises the hormone, acid/alkaline, mineral and water balance.
Bib.: 2 | 4–6 | 8 | 14   **Rarity:** not always available

Diopside, blue
Mineralogy: blue pyroxene mineral (chain silicate, mon., tert.)
Indications: (SP) enfolding of one's personality (S) brings harmony and inner calm (M) helps free oneself from expectations and cope with setbacks (B) fortifies the bladder and kidneys, promotes the function of the sensory organs and nerves.
Bib.: 2 | 4–6 | 8 | 14   **Rarity:** not always available

Diopside 'Star Diopside'
Mineralogy: diopside with asterism (chain silicate, mon., tert.)
Indications: (SP) for spirituality (S) harmonises extreme mood swings (M) aids the recognition of the spiritual nature of being and the underlying spiritual causes of all phenomena (B) fortifies the heart, kidneys, nerves, muscles and blood vessels.
Bib.: 2 | 4–6 | 8 | 14   **Rarity:** scarce

Dioptase
Mineralogy: hydrous copper ring silicate (trig., prim./sec.)
Indications: (SP) for wealth, beauty, happiness (S) helps project oneself in the right light, bestows depth of feeling, hope and intensive dreams (M) helps tap into one's potential, brings a wealth of ideas and creativity (B) fortifies the liver, alleviates pain and cramps.
Bib.: 1 | 2 | 4–6 | 8 | 9 | 12 | 14 | 17   **Rarity:** scarce

Disthene, black
Mineralogy: black aluminium island silicate (tric., tert.)
Indications: (SP) identity, stability (S) strengthens self-assertion, helps overcome extreme lows (M) improves control over one's actions (B) strengthens the kidneys, bladder and nerves, helps with pains, lack of energy and weakness.
Bib.: 4–6 | 8   **Rarity:** not always available

Disthene, blue (Kyanite)
Mineralogy: blue aluminium island silicate (tric., tert.)
Indications: (SP) identity, life-fulfilling vocation (S) helps remain functional in extreme situations (M) promotes a logical way of thinking and resolute action (B) alleviates hoarseness and problems of the larynx; good for the motor nerves and dexterity.
Bib.: 1 | 2 | 4–6 | 8 | 9 | 11 | 14   **Rarity:** not always available

Disthene, green
Mineralogy: green aluminium island silicate (tric., tert.)
Indications: (SP) identity, instinct (S) helps overcome victimhood and resignation (M) overcomes fatalistic attitude and promotes a sure instinctive action (B) alleviates hyperacidity, rheumatism and gout; aids mobility; good for the motor nerves and dexterity.
Bib.: 2 | 4–6 | 8 | 9   **Rarity:** scarce

Disthene, orange
Mineralogy: orange-coloured aluminium island silicate (tric., tert.)
Indications: (SP) optimism, warm-heartedness (S) helps dissipate destructive mind-set and brings a positive attitude to life (M) enables one to recognise the chances presented by each situation (B) boosts the nerves, enhances blood flow and fortifies the muscles.
Bib.: 4   **Rarity:** rare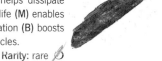

Dolomite, banded (Dolomite Marble)
Mineralogy: dolomite with stripes containing iron (trig., tert.)
Indications: (SP) talent (S) ensures stability and helps with sudden and weighty emotional outbursts (M) aids development of personal abilities (B) alleviates stiff muscles and has a cramp releasing effect, good for the blood, heart, circulation and blood vessels.
Bib.: 1 | 2 | 4–9 | 13 | 14 | 17   **Rarity:** readily available

Dolomite, beige, 'Ivorite'
Mineralogy: calcium magnesium carbonate (trig., sec.)
Indications: (SP) calmness (S) relaxes; lends patience and inner contentment (M) promotes simple pragmatic thinking and helps tackle problems calmly (B) alleviates headaches and reduces deposits in the blood vessels and predisposition to thrombosis.
Bib.: 1 | 2 | 4–7 | 9 | 13 | 14 | 17 | 19   **Rarity:** readily available

Dolomite 'Cobalt Dolomite'

Mineralogy: dolomite containing cobalt (trig., sec.)
Indications: (SP) inspiration, esprit (S) promotes curiosity, imagination and humour (M) lends quick-wittedness, acumen, guile and wit (B) helps with iron deficiency, enhances blood-building, reduces blood pressure and strengthens the thyroid gland, blood vessels, nerves, genitals.
Bib.: 4 | 5   **Rarity:** scarce

Dolomite, orange

Mineralogy: dolomite containing iron (trig., sec./tert.)
Indications: (SP) joy (S) has a restorative and an encouraging effect, stabilises constant mood swings (M) aids discovery of personal abilities (B) stimulates circulation, digestion and metabolism; strengthens the heart in times of great strain.
Bib.: 1 | 2 | 4–6 | 8 | 19   **Rarity:** not always available

Dolomite with Pyrite

Mineralogy: dolomite with pyrite layers (trig./cub., tert.)
Indications: (SP) talent (S) helps convert weaknesses into strengths and redress misunderstandings (M) aids discovery of personal abilities (B) enhances detoxification, de-acidification and excretion; helps with problems of the stomach and intestine.
Bib.: 1 | 2 | 4–7   **Rarity:** readily available

Dolomite, white, 'Sugar Dolomite'

Mineralogy: calcium magnesium carbonate (trig., tert.)
Indications: (SP) self-discovery (S) brings balance and stability (M) enhances common sense; helps achieve personal aims easily and simply (B) relaxes; detoxifies; keeps vital and healthy; relieves pain and releases cramps.
Bib.: 1 | 2 | 4–9 | 13 | 14 | 17 | 19   **Rarity:** readily available

Dumortierite

Mineralogy: aluminium boron silicate (island silicate, rhom., prim.)
Indications: (SP) detachment (S) helps take life lightly and alleviates fear, depression, nervousness and stress (M) helps overcome obsessive behavioural patterns (addiction) (B) alleviates headaches, cramps, diarrhoea, nausea and vomiting.
Bib.: 1–10 | 12–14 | 17   **Rarity:** readily available

Eclipse (Auripigmentum Lime)
Mineralogy: auripigmentum on aragonite (mon./rhom., prim.)
Indications: (SP) impetus, life-affirming (S) enhances the replenishing of life energy after strenuous periods (M) eases letting go of unyielding thoughts and behaviour patterns (B) helps with weak nerves, senses, muscles and inner organs.
Bib.: 4   Rarity: scarce ○

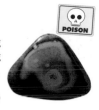

Eclogite
Mineralogy: rock with omphacite and garnet (mon./cub., tert.)
Indications: (SP) recovery (S) brings hope in difficult phases of life; aids the will to recover (M) dissipates fixed ideas of bad luck, danger and failure (B) stimulates regeneration and self-healing power; helps with severe and protracted diseases.
Bib.: 2 | 4 | 6 | 8   **Rarity:** not always available ○

Eilat Stone (Chrysocolla Malachite Azurite)
Mineralogy: mixture of copper minerals (mon., prim./sec.)
Indications: (SP) sense of beauty (S) promotes a lively, eventful and harmonious emotional life (M) gives a fine sense of beauty and harmony (B) fortifies the liver; regulates disharmonious cell growth; alleviates menstrual pains.
Bib.: 2 | 4–6 | 8   **Rarity:** rare ⌀

Eldarite 'Kabamba Stone' (Meta-Rhyolite)
Mineralogy: green stained vulcanite (trig./mon./tric., prim.)
Indications: (SP) self-preservation, immunity, protection (S) protects against external subliminal influences (M) clears doubts and worries (B) supports skin function, sweat glands and body fluids; strengthens the immune system against viral infections.
Bib.: 4 | 5 | 13 | 14 | 17   **Rarity:** readily available ⌀

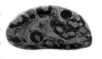

Eldarite 'Nebula stone' (Meta-Rhyolite)
Mineralogy: green stained vulcanite (trig./mon./tric., prim.)
Indications: (SP) integration, vigour, protection (S) overcomes pressure, fear, negativity and external influence (M) clears doubts and worries; brings awareness of suppressed personal interests (B) enhances the function of the skin, sweat glands and body fluids.
Bib.: 4 | 5   **Rarity:** rare ○

Emerald (Beryl)
Mineralogy: beryl containing chromium (ring silicate, hex., prim./tert.)
Indications: (SP) seeking meaning (S) promotes harmony and justice; recuperation and regeneration (M) supports seeking and realising objectives (B) helps with sinusitis, headaches, epilepsy, and diseases of the eyes, heart and intestine.
Bib.: 1–14 | 16 | 17 | 19   **Rarity:** readily available ○

Emerald in Quartzite
Mineralogy: emerald embedded in quartzite matrix (hex./trig., tert.)
Indications: (SP) orientation (S) helps come to terms with blows of fate (M) helps find new orientation in times of crises (B) strengthens the liver, detoxifies, de-acidifies and helps with colds, snoring, infections, inflammations, rheumatism and gout.
Bib.: 1–7 | 17   **Rarity:** not always available ◑

Epidote
Mineralogy: calcium aluminium group silicate (mon., tert.)
Indications: (SP) regeneration (S) brings patience, dissipates anxiety, self-pity and grief (M) helps realise one's idea of happiness and fulfilment (B) fortifies the liver, gallbladder and digestive system; regenerates after over-exertion or illness.
Bib.: 2 | 4–6   **Rarity:** scarce ○

Epidote Feldspar 'Snowflake Epidote'
Mineralogy: rock with epidote and white feldspar (mon., tert.)
Indications: (SP) regeneration (S) helps deal with after-effects of strain or painful experiences (M) teaches not to over-exert oneself (B) fortifies the liver and gallbladder; aids regeneration and recovery, especially when major weaknesses have an obstructive effect.
Bib.: 2 | 4–6   **Rarity:** not always available ○

Epidote Feldspar 'Unakite'
Mineralogy: rock with epidote and pink feldspar (mon., tert.)
Indications: (SP) recovery (S) builds up and strengthens; helps overcome frustrations caused by setbacks (M) teaches not to devalue oneself because of mistakes (B) fortifies the liver and gallbladder; enhances power of regeneration and accelerates healing processes.
Bib.: 1–6 | 8 | 9 | 11 | 13 | 14 | 17   **Rarity:** common ◑

Epidote Quartz

Mineralogy: epidote needles in quartz (trig./mon., tert.)
Indications: (SP) fresh impetus (S) gives courage and hope after great disappointments (M) improves performance and discerning ability (B) rejuvenates quickly; relieves pain and helps with bruises and sprains.
Bib.: 2 | 4–6 | 8   **Rarity:** scarce ○

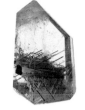

Eudialyte in Syenite

Mineralogy: eudialyte syenite rock (ring silicate, trig., prim.)
Indications: (SP) turning point, new orientation (S) helps overcome grief, fear and pain, accept personal weaknesses (M) for new beginnings, learning from mistakes, overcoming resistance (B) replenishes energy reserves after complete over-exertion.
Bib.: 2 | 4 | 6 | 8   **Rarity:** scarce ○

Falcon's Eye (Fibrous Quartz)

Mineralogy: quartz with crocidolite fibre (trig./mon., sec.)
Indications: (SP) overview, detachment (S) helps with nervousness and inner restlessness (M) makes it easy to retain overview in complex situations and helps with difficulties in decision making (B) relieves pain; helps with shivering, and hormonal hyperactivity.
Bib.: 1 | 2 | 4–6 | 8 | 14 | 17   **Rarity:** common ○

Feldspar 'Multi-coloured Feldspar'

Mineralogy: mixture of different feldspars (mon./tric., prim.)
Indications: (SP) eagerness to learn, new perspective, flexibility (S) feeling of well-being, balance, promotes interest in life itself (M) broadens the perceptive faculty; makes new approaches possible (B) good for spleen, pancreas, stomach, intestine and gallbladder.
Bib.: 2 | 4–6 | 8   **Rarity:** not always available ○

Fire Opal (Precious Opal)

Mineralogy: red/yellow precious opal containing iron (am., prim.)
Indications: (SP) enthusiasm, euphoria (S) makes passionate, very lively and aids enjoyment of sexuality (M) helps one get inspired through challenges (B) boosts the heart, circulation, blood flow, virility and fertility, stimulates the hormonal glands.
Bib.: 1–9 | 11–14 | 17 | 19   **Rarity:** not always available ⚥

Fire Opal (Common Opal)

Mineralogy: red to orange opal containing iron (am., prim.)
Indications: **(SP)** zest for life, enjoyment **(S)** makes impulsive, helps overcome inhibitions, aids enjoyment of sexuality **(M)** awakens enthusiasm for interesting ideas **(B)** enhances energy, performance, circulation, blood flow, virility and fertility.
Bib.: 1–9 | 11–14 | 17 | 19   **Rarity:** not always available ○

Flint (Fire Stone)

Mineralogy: chalcedony and opal mixture (trig./am., sec.)
Indications: **(SP)** for understanding **(S)** calms, for composure **(M)** promotes communicative and listening abilities **(B)** fortifies function of the mucous membranes, lungs, skin and intestine; improves detoxification, helps with constipation and diarrhoea.
Bib.: 2 | 4–6 | 8   **Rarity:** readily available

Fluorite, blue

Mineralogy: calcium fluoride (halide, cub., prim./sec.)
Indications: **(SP)** interest, justice **(S)** makes sober and quiet, helps with frustration and disappointment **(M)** helps give up fixed ideas and aids sense of justice **(B)** alleviates cough and hoarseness; helps with posture damage, adhesions and ganglion.
Bib.: 1–14 | 17 | 19   **Rarity:** readily available

Fluorite, colourless

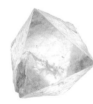

Mineralogy: calcium fluoride (halide, cub., prim./sec.)
Indications: **(SP)** order, purification **(S)** helps with feelings of guilt and impurity, makes more emotionally stable **(M)** clears confusion and helps maintain order **(B)** good for the skin, mucous membranes, respiratory tract, nerves and brain; alleviates cough and allergies.
Bib.: 1–14 | 17 | 19   **Rarity:** readily available ○

Fluorite, green

Mineralogy: calcium fluoride (halogenide, cub., prim.)
Indications: **(SP)** aids creativity and dissolves blockages **(S)** intensifies emotions and moods, making them obvious **(M)** overcomes narrow-mindedness; brings ideas and a quick intellectual grasp **(B)** aids detoxification; helps with arthritis, rheumatism, gout and fungal infections.
Bib.: 1–14 | 17 | 19   **Rarity:** readily available

Fluorite, multi-coloured 'Rainbow fluorite'

Mineralogy: multi-coloured fluorite (halide, cub., prim.)
Indications: (SP) free-thinking spirit, flexibility (S) brings variety and emotional liveliness (M) aids freedom of choice and makes inventive (B) good for the skin, mucous membranes, nerves, bones and teeth; alleviates dry cough, makes joints flexible.
Bib.: 1–14 | 17 | 19   Rarity: readily available

Fluorite, pink

Mineralogy: calcium fluoride (halide, cub., tert.)
Indications: (SP) for goodwill; makes dynamic (S) helps perceive and express suppressed emotions (M) makes active, open and good-natured (B) alleviates functional heart problems; aids hormone regulation; helps with osteoporosis.
Bib.: 1–8 | 19   Rarity: rare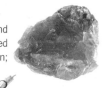

Fluorite, violet

Mineralogy: calcium fluoride (halide, cub., prim./sec.)
Indications: (SP) liberation, self-determination (S) for emotional stability and inner peace (M) helps with learning and concentrating disorders, fortifies the memory (B) helps with overweight caused by wrong eating habits, helps with tumours and septic wounds.
Bib.: 1–14 | 17 | 19   Rarity: readily available ○

Fluorite, yellow

Mineralogy: calcium fluoride (halide, cub., prim./sec.)
Indications: (SP) learning, understanding (S) promotes a positive attitude to life (M) helps digest information and experiences faster (B) helps with stomach problems and eating disorders (including anorexia); fortifies bones and joints.
Bib.: 1–14 | 17 | 19   Rarity: readily available

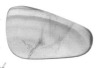

Fuchsite Disthene

Mineralogy: fuchsite and disthene mixture (mon./tric., tert.)
Indications: (SP) integrity, individuality (S) helps remain independent even under pressure; removes fear of losing mental faculties (M) helps avoid injuries (B) helps with roving pain; alleviates inflammations; good for the nerves and skin.
Bib.: 4   Rarity: scarce ○

Fuchsite (Mica)

Mineralogy: chrome mica (sheet silicate, mon., tert.)

Indications: (SP) protection, self-determination **(S)** helps set boundaries; aids a confident appearance **(M)** helps view problems from a distance, thus finding solutions **(B)** helps with allergies, itching, inflammation and effects of radiation.

Bib.: 2 | 4 | 6 | 8 | 9   **Rarity:** readily available ∅

Fulgurite

Mineralogy: sand tube by lightning strike (natural glass, am., tert.)

Indications: (SP) awakening, impetus **(S)** makes elated and free, eases stress, helps quickly pull out of emotional lows **(M)** lends a keen mind and agility in action **(B)** enhances mobility and helps with tendon and ligament injuries.

Bib.: 2 | 4 | 6 | 8   **Rarity:** scarce ○

Gabbro

Mineralogy: mafic intrusive igneous rock (mainly mon./tric., prim.)

Indications: (SP) for new beginnings **(S)** fortifies in times of exhausting routines; aids listening to oneself and perceiving one's needs **(M)** helps plan and prepare new steps carefully **(B)** fortifies the regenerating and self-healing power.

Bib.: 2 | 4 | 6 | 8   **Rarity:** not always available ∅

Galaxyite (Labradorite Rock)

Mineralogy: labradorite/andesine mixture (tric./rhom., prim.)

Indications: (SP) helps emotional depth, striving for fulfilment **(S)** aids deep sleep with good dream recall **(M)** helps constructively combine compassion, clarity and sense of reality **(B)** calms the heartbeat and circulation and aids the function of the kidneys.

Bib.: 2 | 4 | 6 | 8   **Rarity:** scarce ∅

Galena (Lead glance)

Mineralogy: grey lead sulphide (cub., prim./sec./tert.)

Indications: (SP) severity, calm, coming to terms with inner void **(S)** calms disposition, helps overcome melancholy **(M)** turns away thoughts from the past; sobriety **(B)** detoxification; dissolves deposits in the joints; helps with stiffness and immobility.

Bib.: 2 | 4 | 6 | 8   **Rarity:** readily available ∅

Garnet Amphibolite

Mineralogy: almandine in amphibolite (cub./mon./tric., tert.)
Indications: (SP) conclude, bring to an end **(S)** helps transform causes of discord **(M)** promotes pragmatic thinking and unswerving action **(B)** helps with nervous heart problems and constrictions, boosts circulation, the kidneys, metabolism and digestion.
Bib.: 4   **Rarity:** scarce ○

Garnet Mica Schist

Mineralogy: almandine in mica schist (cub./mon., tert.)
Indications: (SP) willpower, fitness, capacity for work **(S)** gives strength to master great difficulties **(M)** gives vigour to carry out ideas and duties **(B)** boosts performance, stimulates metabolism and promotes detoxification and excretion at the same time.
Bib.: 1 | 2 | 6 | 8   **Rarity:** readily available ⌀

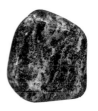

Garnet Peridotite (Olivine Garnet Rock)

Mineralogy: pyrope in meta-peridotite (cub./rhom., tert.)
Indications: (SP) stubbornness, unyielding nature **(S)** helps remain faithful to oneself amid great adjustment pressure **(M)** makes more determined to stand up for one's convictions **(B)** for elasticity, boosts circulation, liver, bile, nerves, tendons, muscles and joints.
Bib.: 4   **Rarity:** scarce ⌀

Garnet Pyroxenite

Mineralogy: almandine in pyroxenite (cub./rhom./mon., tert.)
Indications: (SP) self-assertion, perseverance **(S)** strengthens the will to live, helps with strain and exhaustion **(M)** urges to tackle what is necessary with vigour **(B)** boots digestion, stabilises circulation and strengthens the muscles.
Bib.: 4   **Rarity:** scarce ⌀

Gaspeite

Mineralogy: iron and magnesium nickel carbonate (trig., sec.)
Indications: (SP) life-affirming **(S)** peps up, makes jovial, aids benevolence and agility **(M)** self-critical, makes quick-witted enough to recognise pranks played by self or others **(B)** helpful for detoxification and over-acidity (with chalcedony for elimination).
Bib.: 2 | 4 | 6 | 8   **Rarity:** scarce ⌀

Green Quartz (Fuchsite Quartzite)

Mineralogy: green quartz containing fuchsite (trig./mon., tert.)
Indications: (SP) for appeasement (S) helps with adjustment and inner turmoil, relieves stress (M) enables calm, prudent reflection (B) strengthens the liver, eases gallbladder problems, helps with rheumatism, inflammations, rashes and sunburns.
Bib.: 4 | 19   **Rarity:** common ○

Grossular, green (Garnet)

Mineralogy: green calcium aluminium island silicate (cub., tert.)
Indications: (SP) restorative; regeneration (S) brings hope and optimism in difficult phases of life (M) helps develop new perspectives (B) fortifies liver and kidney; helps with rheumatism and arthritis; detoxifies and regenerates the skin and mucous membranes.
Bib.: 1 | 2 | 4–6 | 8 | 14 | 19   **Rarity:** not always available ∅

Grossular, pink (Garnet)

Mineralogy: pink calcium aluminium island silicate (cub., tert.)
Indications: (SP) vitalisation, regeneration (S) promotes willingness to indulge in mutual help (M) helps harmonise ideals with reality (B) strengthens the heart, circulation, liver and kidneys, enhances blood circulation, detoxification and regenerates the skin and mucous membranes.
Bib.: 1 | 2 | 4–6 | 8 | 14 | 19   **Rarity:** not always available ∅

Grossularite (Garnet)

Mineralogy: rock containing grossular (mostly cub., tert.)
Indications: (SP) restorative; fosters community spirit (S) promotes social unity in difficult times (M) helps formulate new ideas and express them (B) fortifies the liver and kidneys; helps with rheumatism and arthritis; detoxifies and regenerates the skin and mucous membranes.
Bib.: 1 | 2 | 4 | 6 | 8 | 14   **Rarity:** not always available ∅

Halite, blue (Salt Stone)

Mineralogy: blue sodium chloride (halide, cub., sec.)
Indications: (SP) for clarity, cleansing (S) brings inner calm, helps with stress, protects against attacks on one's aura (M) ends pondering and listlessness, boosts concentration (B) cleanses and detoxifies, alleviates allergies, asthma and autoimmune diseases.
Bib.: 2 | 4–6 | 15   **Rarity:** scarce ○

Halite, colourless (Salt Stone, Salt Crystal)

Mineralogy: pure sodium chloride (halide, cub., sec.)
Indications: (SP) liberation, purification (S) makes lively and brings inner balance (M) dissolves unconscious thought and behavioural patterns (B) regulates metabolism and water balance; eliminates, detoxifies, cleanses and protects the respiratory tract, intestine and skin.
Bib.: 2 | 4–6 | 8–10 | 14 | 15　　　　　**Rarity:** common ○

Halite, orange (Salt Stone)

Mineralogy: orange sodium chloride (halide, cub., sec.)
Indications: (SP) for protection, cleansing (S) helps with worries and fear, improves quality of life (M) strengthens decision-making power (B) cleanses, purifies, detoxifies, strengthens the connective tissues and skin, boosts digestion and improves absorption of nutrients.
Bib.: 2 | 4–6 | 8–10 | 14 | 15　　　　　**Rarity:** common ⵁ

Halite, pink (Salt Stone)

Mineralogy: pink sodium chloride (halide, cub., sec.)
Indications: (SP) eases burden, cleansing (S) promotes a life-affirming attitude and lightens mood (M) helps free one's attention from the past (B) purifies, detoxifies, helps with colds and inflammations.
Bib.: 2 | 4–6 | 8–10 | 14 | 15　　　**Rarity:** readily available ⵁ

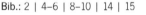
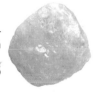

Halite, purple (Salt Stone)

Mineralogy: purple sodium chloride (halide, cub., sec.)
Indications: (SP) for letting go, cleansing (S) eases grief, worries, old sufferings and resignation (M) helps with concentration problems and confusion (B) purifies, detoxifies, cleanses the lymph, intestine and skin and helps with diseases of the thyroid gland and respiratory tract.
Bib.: 2 | 4–6 | 15　　　　　　　　**Rarity:** scarce ○

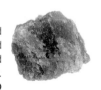

Hauyne

Mineralogy: blue aluminium silicate (lattice silicate, cub., prim.)
Indications: (SP) consciousness, recognition (S) frees from attachments, compulsions and negative emotions (M) enables deep understanding and helps get to the heart of things (B) clears nostrils and sinuses, improves perception of the body.
Bib.: 2 | 4 | 6　　　　　　　　　　**Rarity:** rare ○

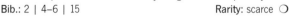
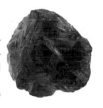

Heliodor (Beryl)
Mineralogy: yellowish green beryl (ring silicate, hex., prim.)
Indications: (SP) resistance, stability (S) helps bear immense pressure (internal and external); reduces aggressiveness (M) helps plan in advance while still remaining flexible (B) strengthens the immune system and helps with short- and long-sightedness.
Bib.: 1 | 2 | 4 | 5 | 6 | 8 **Rarity:** scarce ○

Heliotrope (Chalcedony)
Mineralogy: green chalcedony with red spots (trig., prim.)
Indications: (SP) immune protection (S) aids setting boundaries (M) helps maintain control (B) fortifies the lymph and immune reaction; helps with problems of the heart, blood vessels and bladder as well as with 'flu, colds, infections, inflammation and pus formation.
Bib.: 1–14 | 16–18 **Rarity:** common ○

Hematite
Mineralogy: iron oxide (trig., sec./tert.)
Indications: (SP) survival (S) promotes striving for improvement of one's situation in life (M) helps pursue aims with determination and to fight for them if necessary (B) aids assimilation of iron, blood-building, circulation and blood flow, fortifies the muscles and kidneys.
Bib.: 1–6 | 8–12 | 14 | 17 | 19 **Rarity:** not always available

Hematite, banded (Banded Iron Ore)
Mineralogy: iron oxide (trig., sec. or tert. iron ore)
Indications: (SP) strength, endurance (S) fortifies staying power during intensive work or exertion (M) helps realise one's plans in spite of obstacles (B) promotes iron assimilation, blood-building and oxygen transport; fortifies the liver, spleen and intestine.
Bib.: 2–6 | 8 | 14 | 17 **Rarity:** not always available

Hematite (Kidney Ore)
Mineralogy: iron oxide (trig., as kidney ore prim.)
Indications: (SP) improvement (S) fortifies willpower and brings unfulfilled wishes to light (M) directs attention to basic needs and physical well-being (B) promotes iron assimilation and blood-building; fortifies the small and large intestines and kidneys.
Bib.: 1–6 | 8 | 10–12 | 14 | 19 **Rarity:** not always available

Hematite with Magnetite

Mineralogy: iron oxide (trig./cub., tert. iron ore)
Indications: (SP) progress, engagement (S) brings vitality, energy and dynamism into life (M) mirrors one's inner outlook and views (B) aids assimilation of iron and blood-building, stimulates the glands, liver and gallbladder.
Bib.: 2–6 | 8–12 | 14 | 17 | 19   **Rarity:** common

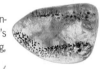

Hematite Quartz

Mineralogy: hematite platelets in crystal quartz (trig., prim./sec./tert.)
Indications: (SP) vitality (S) strengthens, rejuvenates, cheers up, enhances courage and enthusiasm (M) helps properly apportion one's energy in spiritual and physical exertions (B) enhances blood-building, stabilises circulation, fortifies the muscles, nerves and senses.
Bib.: 2 | 4–6 | 8   **Rarity:** not always available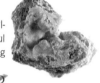

Hemimorphite, blue

Mineralogy: zinc group silicate containing copper (rhom., sec.)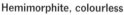
Indications: (SP) spiritual advancement (S) promotes sexual fulfilment and a calm, peaceful disposition (M) harmonises mind and soul (B) helps with skin problems, warts, sunburn and burns, wound healing and restless legs.
Bib.: 2 | 4–6 | 8   **Rarity:** scarce

Hemimorphite, colourless

Mineralogy: alkaline zinc group silicate (rhom., sec.)
Indications: (SP) helps focus on one's goal (S) has an emotionally uplifting effect and brings new impetus (M) helps recognise external influences (B) boosts the brain nerves and immune reaction, enhances wound healing and helps with restless legs.
Bib.: 2 | 4–6 | 8   **Rarity:** scarce ○

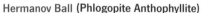

Hermanov Ball (Phlogopite Anthophyllite)

Mineralogy: phlogopite in anthophyllite (mon./rhom., tert.)
Indications: (SP) trust, innocence, protection (S) bestows a positive disposition to life, helps retain a soft core under an external hard shell (M) ends self-doubt and agonising brooding (B) detoxifies and regulates the function of the kidneys and gonads.
Bib.: 2 | 4–6 | 8   **Rarity:** rare ○

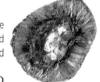

Hessonite (Garnet)

Mineralogy: grossular containing iron (island silicate, cub., tert.)
Indications: **(SP)** self-respect; restorative; growth **(S)** soothes emotional agitation, brings clarity into emotions **(M)** helps appreciate one's abilities **(B)** fortifies the liver and kidneys; regulates hormone balance in cases of hyper and hypo function of glands.
Bib.: 1 | 2 | 4–6 | 8 | 19   **Rarity:** scarce

Heulandite

Mineralogy: zeolite leaves (lattice silicate, mon. prim./sec./tert.)
Indications: **(SP)** mobility **(S)** helps let go of negative emotions **(M)** makes changing habits easier **(B)** fortifies the kidneys and liver; promotes blood flow; good for mobility, joints, discs, meniscus (knee) and feet.
Bib.: 2 | 4–6 | 8   **Rarity:** not always available

Hiddenite (Spodumene)

Mineralogy: yellowish-green chain silicate (pyroxene, mon./prim.)
Indications: **(SP)** devotion **(S)** teaches devotion without self-denial **(M)** improves memory, helps with difficulties in decision making **(B)** alleviates problems of the joints; helps with nervous diseases, neuralgia, sciatic neuralgia and toothache.
Bib.: 2 | 4–6 | 8 | 19   **Rarity:** scarce ○

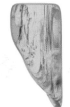

Hilutite (Garnet Zircon Quartz)

Mineralogy: quartz with garnet and zircon (trig./cub./tetr., prim.)
Indications: **(SP)** for presence of mind, purpose in life **(S)** lends life-affirming disposition, promotes social contact, has a sexually arousing effect **(M)** structures thinking, enables constructive resolution of conflicts **(B)** stimulates healing process for chronic ailments.
Bib.: 4 | 6   **Rarity:** scarce ○

Hornblende

Mineralogy: amphibole (chain silicate, mon., prim./tert.)
Indications: **(SP)** unity, integration **(S)** helps dissipate inner conflict and obsessive tension **(M)** helps cope with disparities by allowing each aspect its necessary space **(B)** good for the small intestine and kidneys as well as for middle and inner ear problems.
Bib.: 2 | 4 | 6 | 8   **Rarity:** scarce ○

Howlite

Mineralogy: calcium boron silicate (island silicate, mon., sec.)
Indications: (SP) independence, mindfulness **(S)** aids taking control of one's life **(M)** promotes conscious control of one's actions **(B)** fortifies sense of balance; helps with nausea, eases vomiting; ameliorates skin irritation caused by contact poison.
Bib.: 2 | 4–6 | 8 | 19   Rarity: scarce

Hydrogrossular (Garnet)

Mineralogy: grossularite containing hydroxide (island silicate, cub., tert.)
Indications: (SP) restorative; helps amendment, order **(S)** brings emotional engagement, dissipates self-pity **(M)** replaces wrong ideas with a realistic view **(B)** fortifies the kidneys, liver and gallbladder; aids detoxification and elimination.
Bib.: 4 | 6 | 8 | 14 | 19   Rarity: scarce

Hypersthene (Ferro-Enstatite)

Mineralogy: glittering chain silicate (pyroxene, rhom., prim.)
Indications: (SP) balance **(S)** brings right measure of activity and rest; makes dynamic and emotionally balanced **(M)** helps accept criticism and defend one's conviction **(B)** eases tension, relieves pain and helps with hyperacidity.
Bib.: 2 | 4–6 | 8   Rarity: scarce

Ilmenite Quartz

Mineralogy: ilmenite needles in quartz (oxide, trig., prim.)
Indications: (SP) inspiration, image **(S)** accentuates personality, character and abilities **(M)** helps differentiate between inspiration and illusion and to attempt great deeds **(B)** helps with signs of constriction, degeneration or wear and tear.
Bib.: 2 | 4 | 6   Rarity: rare

Iron Quartz (Quartz)

Mineralogy: crystal quartz containing iron (trig., prim./sec./tert.)
Indications: (SP) energy **(S)** mobilises emotional and physical energy reserves, brings vigour **(M)** helps pursue envisaged plans energetically **(B)** improves performance; stimulates circulation and blood flow; fortifies blood vessels and muscles.
Bib.: 2 | 4 | 6 | 8   Rarity: not always available

Iron Nickel Meteorite
Mineralogy: iron nickel alloy (cub., interplanetary formation)
Indications: (SP) aids cross-checking personal intentions and aims **(S)** releases inner images, renews outdated structures **(M)** helps accept new perspectives, question existing values and energetically materialise spontaneous impulses **(B)** regulates muscle tension.
Bib.: 2 | 4–6 | 8   **Rarity:** readily available ◯

Jadeite, 'Jade'
Mineralogy: chain silicate of the pyroxene group (mon., tert.)
Indications: (SP) balance **(S)** maintains balance between work and rest **(M)** aids self-realisation with great ease **(B)** regulates the nerves, kidneys and adrenal glands (adrenaline production); maintains water, mineral and acid-base balance.
Bib.: 1 | 2 | 4–9 | 14 | 19   **Rarity:** not always available ◑

Jadeite, black, 'Jade black'
Mineralogy: black jadeite (chain silicate, mon., tert.)
Indications: (SP) right measure **(S)** frees from negative emotions, calms and consolidates **(M)** helps remain neutral and find the right balance in one's activity **(B)** regulates elimination and excretion through the kidneys and bladder.
Bib.: 4 | 6 | 19   **Rarity:** scarce ◑

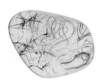

Jamesonite Quartz
Mineralogy: jamesonite in quartz (mon./trig., prim./tert.)
Indications: (SP) subordination **(S)** bestows discipline to overcome negative habits **(M)** helps place personal interests below higher ideals **(B)** helps with weak immunity as well as with problems of the bones, skin and nerves; enhances detoxification.
Bib.: 2 | 4 | 6   **Rarity:** rare ∅

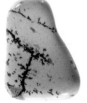

Jasper, beige 'Ivory Jasper'
Mineralogy: ivory-coloured jasper (quartz, trig., prim.)
Indications: (SP) cleansing **(S)** brings constant, harmonious flow of power, helps avoid extremes **(M)** eases letting go of external thoughts **(B)** has a strong purifying effect; cleanses the connective tissues; alleviates allergies and skin problems.
Bib.: 2 | 4 | 5 | 8 | 11 | 17   **Rarity:** readily available ◯

Jasper, beige-brown 'Cappuccino Jasper'
Mineralogy: cappuccino-coloured jasper (quartz, trig., prim.)
Indications: (SP) performance (S) bestows stability, promotes inner calm (M) helps tackle a huge pile of work by sensibly apportioning one's energy (B) fortifies the stomach, intestine and immune system; promotes cleansing and elimination.
Bib.: 2 | 4 | 5 | 8 | 11 | 17   **Rarity:** readily available

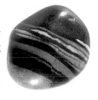

Jasper 'Breccia Jasper', 'Brecciated Jasper'
Mineralogy: breccia jasper with chalcedony sealing (trig., sec.)
Indications: (SP) makes ready for conflicts (S) helps to stand up again and again after defeats (M) eases resolution of conflicts and helps make up for harm (B) rejuvenates and vitalises; stimulates circulation, blood flow and self-healing power.
Bib.: 1 | 2 | 4–6 | 8 | 11 | 13 | 14 | 16 | 17 **Rarity:** common ○

Jasper, brownish-grey 'Picture Jasper'
Mineralogy: Jasper with picturesque illustrations (trig., prim.)
Indications: (SP) helps come to terms with situations (S) helps bear energy-sapping situations in life (M) brings joy in simple things (B) enhances cleansing and purification of the connective tissues, stimulates elimination and alleviates allergic reactions.
Bib.: 2 | 4–6 | 8 | 11 | 17   **Rarity:** readily available ○

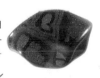

Jasper, brown
Mineralogy: jasper in different shades of brown (trig., prim.)
Indications: (SP) untiring (S) promotes stability, perseverance and flexibility (when necessary) (M) helps drive ongoing projects with determination (B) stimulates digestion and elimination; stabilises circulation and helps with deep exhaustion.
Bib.: 2 | 4–6 | 8 | 11 | 17 | 19   **Rarity:** readily available

Jasper, coloured
Mineralogy: multi-coloured jasper (quartz, trig., prim./sec.)
Indications: (SP) creative power (S) rejuvenates and brings an active emotional life (M) supports creative realisation of one's ideas (B) enhances detoxification and the immune system; regenerates the functional tissue of organs (parenchyma).
Bib.: 1 | 2 | 4–6 | 8 | 12 | 16 | 17 | 19   **Rarity:** readily available

Jasper, green
Mineralogy: jasper containing iron silicate (quartz, trig., prim.)
Indications: (SP) for resistance and harmony (S) calms emotions, helps express and accept them (M) improves control over thoughts and actions (B) fortifies the immune system, helps with 'flu, colds, infections and inflammation.
Bib.: 1 | 2 | 4–6 | 8 | 9 | 16 | 17 | 19   **Rarity:** readily available ○

Jasper with Hematite, 'Iron Jasper'
Mineralogy: mixture of jasper and hematite (oxide, trig., tert.)
Indications: (SP) fitness (S) increases stamina under heavy strain (M) helps achieve and follow through one's ideas skilfully and emphatically (B) improves iron absorption and formation of red blood cells; stimulates circulation and blood flow.
Bib.: 1 | 2 | 4–6 | 8 | 11 | 13 | 14 | 17   **Rarity:** not always available ∅

Jasper 'Poppy Jasper'
Mineralogy: colourfully patterned jasper (quartz, trig., sec.)
Indications: (SP) mood-enhancing (S) brings cheerfulness, gives impetus for variety and new experiences (M) stimulates imagination and versatility thus also helping to realise ideas (B) enhances the immune system, liver, circulation and regenerative powers.
Bib.: 1 | 2 | 4–6 | 8 | 16 | 17   **Rarity:** readily available ○

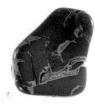

Jasper, red
Mineralogy: jasper containing hematite (quartz, trig., sec.)
Indications: (SP) willpower (S) makes courageous, dynamic; gives energy and enhances warrior-nature (M) gives courage for unpleasant tasks and makes spiritually alert (B) warms and enlivens; enhances blood flow, stimulates blood circulation and has a fever-enhancing effect.
Bib.: 1– 6 | 8 | 9 | 11–14 | 16 | 17 | 19   **Rarity:** common ∅

Jasper 'Turitella Jasper'
Mineralogy: fossilised snail shells (jasper, trig., sec.-prim.)
Indications: (SP) withdrawal (S) helps overcome feelings of guilt (M) reminds one of one's wishes, goals and plans (B) enhances detoxification and elimination; increases resistance against environmental pollution (grime, toxins, radiation).
Bib.: 1 | 2 | 4–6 | 8 | 11 | 17   **Rarity:** common ∅

Jasper 'Vulcano Jasper'
Mineralogy: breccia with jasper in chalcedony (trig., sec.)
Indications: **(SP)** alertness, caution **(S)** enhances one's sixth sense for dangers **(M)** helps act calmly, quickly and resolutely in critical situations **(B)** stimulates cleansing of the connective tissues, lymph and blood; activates the spleen, liver, kidneys and intestine.
Bib.: 2 | 4 | 6 | 8   **Rarity:** readily available

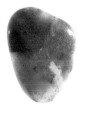

Jasper, yellow
Mineralogy: jasper containing limonite (quartz, trig., sec.)
Indications: **(SP)** endurance **(S)** promotes perseverance and tenacity **(M)** helps digest experiences and endure frustrating experiences **(B)** builds up a stable long-term immune protection; aids digestion; purifies and firms up the connective tissues.
Bib.: 1 | 2 | 4–9 | 11 | 16 | 17 | 19   **Rarity:** readily available

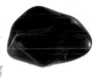

Jet (Gagate, Lignite, Brown Coal)
Mineralogy: carbon rock rich in bitumen (am., sec.)
Indications: **(SP)** hope **(S)** helps overcome anxiety and depression **(M)** aids working on positive changes in a robust, unrelenting and persevering manner **(B)** helps with problems of the mouth, gum, intestine (diarrhoea), skin, joints and spine.
Bib.: 2–6 | 8 | 9 | 11 | 14 | 17   **Rarity:** readily available

Kalahari Picture Stone (Landscape stone)
Mineralogy: sandstone quartz (trig., sec.)
Indications: **(SP)** staying power **(S)** strengthens under prolonged strain **(M)** helps to try again constantly, even after failing **(B)** aids digestion, the immune system and cleansing of the connective tissues and so alleviates allergies and hay fever.
Bib.: 2 | 4–6 | 8 | 11 | 13 | 14 | 17   **Rarity:** common ○

Kimberlite
Mineralogy: volcano breccia (mainly mon./rhom., prim.)
Indications: **(SP)** transformation **(S)** eases painful processes in life and gives new zeal **(M)** helps give up resistance against change and unites irreconcilables **(B)** promotes de-acidification and regulates the mineral balance in the body.
Bib.: 2 | 4 | 8   **Rarity:** not always available

Kunzite (Spodumene)

Mineralogy: pink chain silicate (pyroxene group, mon., prim.)
Indications: (SP) humility **(S)** improves empathy, helps with difficulties in making contact **(M)** helps accept criticism, promotes tolerance and readiness to serve **(B)** helps with neuralgia, sciatic neuralgia and toothache; releases tension in the heart region.
Bib.: 1–14 | 17 | 19   **Rarity:** not always available ○

Labradorite (Feldspar)

Mineralogy: coloured glittering feldspar (lattice silicate, tric., prim.)
Indications: (SP) reflection, truth **(S)** sharpens intuition, promotes emotional depth and mediumistic abilities **(M)** brings forgotten memories to light and helps recognise illusions **(B)** reduces sensitivity to cold and blood pressure and alleviates rheumatism and gout.
Bib.: 1–10 | 11–14 | 17   **Rarity:** readily available ⬭

Labradorite 'Gold Labradorite' (Feldspar)

Mineralogy: yellowish gold labradorite (lattice silicate, tric., prim.)
Indications: (SP) esteem **(S)** promotes self-confidence, helps with distrust and fears **(M)** enables assessing the value and importance of a situation **(B)** enhances energy distribution in the body, strengthens the spleen, pancreas and the vegetative nervous system.
Bib.: 2 | 4 | 5   **Rarity:** not always available ⬭

Labradorite 'Spectrolite' (Feldspar)

Mineralogy: very colourful labradorite (lattice silicate, tric., prim.)
Indications: (SP) imagination, creativity **(S)** enhances artistic talents and a keen sense for harmonious connections **(M)** makes enthusiastic, imaginative and creative **(B)** reduces sensitivity to cold; alleviates rheumatism and gout.
Bib.: 1–14 | 17   **Rarity:** not always available ⬭

Labradorite, white 'Rainbow Moonstone' (Feldspar)

Mineralogy: blue shining white labradorite (tric., prim.)
Indications: (SP) sensitivity **(S)** improves perceptive faculty, sleep and dream recall **(M)** promotes alertness and power of observation **(B)** improves sense of well-being; regulates the female hormonal cycle and helps with menstrual pains.
Bib.: 2 | 4–6 | 8 | 14 | 19   **Rarity:** readily available ○

Lapis Lazuli

Mineralogy: lasurite rock (lasurite: lattice silicate, cub., tert.)
Indications: **(SP)** truth **(S)** promotes honesty, dignity, friendship and sociability **(M)** helps tell and accept the truth **(B)** helps with problems of the throat, larynx, vocal cords, nerves and brain; regulates the thyroid gland.
Bib.: 1–14 | 16 | 17 | 19   **Rarity:** readily available

Lapis Lazuli with Calcite 'Spotted Lapis'

Mineralogy: mixture of lapis lazuli and calcite (cub./trig., tert.)
Indications: **(SP)** enhances sense of personal responsibility **(S)** promotes genuineness and helps gain control over one's life **(M)** enhances power of discernment and intelligence; helps open up to others **(B)** reduces fever and blood pressure; slows down the menstrual cycle.
Bib.: 1–8 | 11 | 12 | 14 | 16 | 17 | 19   **Rarity:** readily available ○

Larimar (blue Pectolite)

Mineralogy: blue pectolite (chain silicate, tric., prim.)
Indications: **(SP)** promotes openness **(S)** helps increase and demarcate spiritual space as well as digest absorbed impressions **(M)** broadens sense of perception **(B)** stimulates brain activity and sensitivity; helps with problems of the chest, throat and head.
Bib.: 1 | 2 | 4–6 | 8 | 9 | 12 | 14 | 19 **Rarity:** not always available ○

Larvikite (Syenite Monzonite)

Mineralogy: magmatite rich in feldspar (tric./mon./trig., prim.)
Indications: **(SP)** promotes clear assessment, straightforwardness **(S)** reduces emotions, makes sober and neutral **(M)** helps understand and resolve complicated facts **(B)** purifies the tissues, calms the nerves, cools and reduces blood pressure.
Bib.: 2 | 4 | 8 | 17   **Rarity:** readily available ○

Lava (Vesicular Basalt)

Mineralogy: porous basalt (mon./tric., prim.)
Indications: **(SP)** movement **(S)** promotes self-perception and awareness of one's well-being, condition **(M)** makes determined and protects against negligence and hollow compromises **(B)** relaxes the organs of the lower abdomen, eases stiff muscles and warms the limbs.
Bib.: 2 | 4 | 6 | 8   **Rarity:** readily available

Lavender Jade (purple Jadeite)
Mineralogy: jadeite containing manganese (chain silicate, mon., tert.)
Indications: (SP) inner peace (S) brings inner harmony, eases nervousness and irritability (M) helps overcome disappointments and resolve conflicts in relationships (B) helps kidney problems; alleviates inflammation, pains in the heart and nerves; toothache.
Bib.: 1–6 | 8 | 19　　　　　　　　　　**Rarity:** scarce

Lavender Quartz (purple Chalcedony)
Mineralogy: lavender coloured chalcedony (trig., prim./sec.)
Indications: (SP) understanding, sensitivity (S) combines calmness and attentiveness; makes sensitive to the needs of others (M) enhances understanding and readiness to continuously learn (B) fortifies the kidneys and secretion of the glands; reduces blood pressure.
Bib.: 2 | 4 | 5 | 8　　　　　　　　**Rarity:** not always available ○

Lazulite
Mineralogy: alkaline aluminium phosphate (mon., sec./tert.)
Indications: (SP) spiritual orientation (S) makes emotions and feelings more obvious, bestows peace (M) aids reflection on meaning, value and importance of life (B) fortifies and relaxes; gently regulates the nerves, metabolism and hormonal system.
Bib.: 2 | 4 | 6 | 8　　　　　　　　　**Rarity:** rare ⌀

Lepidolite (Mica)
Mineralogy: lithium mica (sheet silicate, mon., prim.)
Indications: (SP) sets boundaries (S) protects against external influences; gives inner peace; helps with sleep disorders (M) frees from distractions, helps concentrate on important aspects (B) alleviates pains in the joints and nerves, sciatica and neuralgia.
Bib.: 1 | 2 | 4–6 | 8 | 9　　　　　　**Rarity:** readily available ○

Lemon Chrysoprase (Nickel Magnesite, Citron Chrysoprase')
Mineralogy: magnesia containing nickel partly silicified (trig., sec.)
Indications: (SP) life-affirming, frankness (S) cheers, helps overcome loneliness and inhibitions (M) makes self-critical, funny and clever (B) helpful for cleansing, for hyperacidity as well as stiff muscles and the effects of over-exertion.
Bib.: 2 | 4–6 | 8 | 19　　　　　　**Rarity:** not always available ⌀

Libyan Desert Glass (Natural Glass)
Mineralogy: solidified silicon dioxide molten glass (am., prim.)
Indications: (SP) cheerfulness, fun **(S)** makes spontaneous, impulsive and sociable, gives joie de vivre **(M)** helps release doubts and allow diverse views **(B)** helps with clouding of the eyeball and lenses (cataracts); good for the stomach and pancreas.
Bib.: 2 | 4 | 6   **Rarity:** scarce ○

Limonite (Clay Ironstone)
Mineralogy: limonite rock (iron oxide, rhom., sec.)
Indications: (SP) promotes inner strength **(S)** gives strength under extreme strain; helps convert selfishness to a sense of community **(M)** helps remain firm in the face of attacks without fighting back **(B)** promotes cleansing; aids digestion and elimination.
Bib.: 2 | 4 | 6 | 8   **Rarity:** readily available ∅

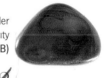

Lizardite (Serpentine)
Mineralogy: alkaline magnesium sheet silicate (trig., tert.)
Indications: (SP) gratitude **(S)** makes happy and lends the feeling of being carried through life **(M)** enables amicable resolution of conflicts and reconciliation **(B)** detoxifies, eases over-acidity, helps with cramps, good for the liver, gallbladder, kidneys and digestion.
Bib.: 4 | 5 | 19   **Rarity:** not always available ∅

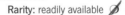

Magnesite (compact)
Mineralogy: magnesium carbonate (trig., sec./tert.)
Indications: (SP) relaxes **(S)** makes patient; helps with nervousness, bashfulness and irritability **(M)** promotes the art of listening **(B)** helps with migraine, headaches, cramps, colic and tension; guards against deposits in the vessels and heart attack.
Bib.: 1–11 | 13 | 14 | 17–19   **Rarity:** common ∅

Magnesite (nodule)
Mineralogy: magnesium carbonate (trig., sec.)
Indications: (SP) flexibility **(S)** helps become more flexible, without giving up one's plans; eases stress **(M)** promotes the ability to simply allow things to take their normal course instead of making a huge effort **(B)** detoxifies, de-acidifies, eases strain and cramps.
Bib.: 1–11 | 13 | 14 | 17–19   **Rarity:** readily available ∅

Magnetite
Mineralogy: magnetic iron oxide (cub., prim./tert.)
Indications: (SP) for activation and orientation **(S)** increases reflex action **(M)** stimulates aiming for higher ideals; helps differentiate between useful and useless things **(B)** stimulates energy flow and activities of the glands; activates the liver and bile production.
Bib.: 2 | 4–6 | 8 | 9 | 14 | 16 | 19   **Rarity:** readily available

Malachite
Mineralogy: alkaline copper carbonate (mon., prim./sec.)
Indications: (SP) promotes adventurous intensive life **(S)** deepens emotional life, helps with sexual difficulties **(M)** promotes power of imagination and decision **(B)** stimulates the brain, nerves and liver, detoxifies and helps with rheumatism, cramps and menstrual pains.
Bib.: 1–14 | 17 | 19   **Rarity:** readily available ○

Marble (Calcite Marble)
Mineralogy: metamorphic lime (calcium carbonate, trig., tert.)
Indications: (SP) aids transformation **(S)** changes inner discontentment and unhappy life circumstances **(M)** opens up new perspectives, brings creative solutions to problems **(B)** enhances the development of children; fortifies the kidneys and spleen; alleviates allergies.
Bib.: 1 | 2 | 4 | 6 | 8 | 19   **Rarity:** readily available ⌀

Marble 'Zebra Marble' (Dolomite Marble)
Mineralogy: metamorphic dolomite with manganese (trig., tert.)
Indications: (SP) self-liberation **(S)** helps defend oneself against suppression, improves constant discontentment **(M)** helps overcome resignation **(B)** promotes cleansing and elimination; eases allergies; fortifies the spleen, kidneys, intestine, tissues and skin.
Bib.: 1 | 2 | 4 | 6 | 8 | 19   **Rarity:** readily available ⌀

Marcasite
Mineralogy: iron sulphide (rhom., prim./sec.)
Indications: (SP) for self-worth **(S)** helps appreciate oneself and brings suppressed desires to light **(M)** helps to find the causes of one's unhappiness and to give up compliant and subservient behaviours **(B)** stimulates detoxification and elimination.
Bib.: 2 | 4 | 6 | 8   **Rarity:** not always available ⌀

Maw-Sit-Sit

Mineralogy: rock with jadeite, albite, chlorite a.o. (mon./tric. a.o., tert.)
Indications: (SP) for balance, tolerance, carefulness **(S)** cures bad-temperedness, promotes well-being and trust **(M)** helps accept the unchangeable **(B)** relieves pain; strengthens the nerves; gives new energy and vitality; helps with kidney problems.
Bib.: 2 | 4 | 6 | 8 | 19

Rarity: scarce ○

Melanite (Garnet)

Mineralogy: Andradite containing titanium (island silicate, cub., tert.)
Indications: (SP) self-discovery, sincerity **(S)** for reliability, stability and trust **(M)** makes more receptive to one's conscience and strengthens 'resistance' in disputes **(B)** promotes growth in height and fortifies the bones and spine.
Bib.: 1 | 2 | 4 | 6 | 8 | 19

Rarity: scarce ◑

Metagabbro

Mineralogy: metamorphically transformed gabbro (mon./tric., tert.)
Indications: (SP) gives overview, instinct **(S)** helps become clear of one's feelings **(M)** enhances trusting in one's inner voice and observing the consequences of one's deeds **(B)** strengthens the nerves, kidneys and digestion, good for the ears, larynx and voice.
Bib.: 4

Rarity: scarce ◐

Meta-Rhyolite 'Rainforest Stone'

Mineralogy: silicified vulcanite (trig./mon./tric./am., prim.)
Indications: (SP) intensification **(S)** consolidates existing circumstances; helps accept oneself as one is **(M)** helps see and assess one's situation more clearly **(B)** alleviates 'flu, colds and infections.
Bib.: 1 | 2 | 4–6 | 8 | 17

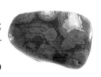

Rarity: readily available ○

Meta-Rhyolite 'Dr. Liesegang Stone', 'Aztec Stone'

Mineralogy: silicified vulcanite (trig./mon./tric./am., prim.)
Indications: (SP) fortification **(S)** consolidates existing circumstances; promotes self-esteem **(M)** helps master hard situations calmly and resolutely **(B)** enhances resistance and the immune system; stimulates the small and large intestines.
Bib.: 2 | 4–6 | 8

Rarity: not always available ◐

Meta-Rhyolite 'Leopard stone'
Mineralogy: silicified vulcanite (trig./mon./tric./am., prim.)
Indications: (SP) consolidation (S) for balance between activity and rest, good for deep sleep (M) makes clear what needs to be done – without new impulse (B) stimulates digestion and excretion; helps with skin problems and hardened tissues.
Bib.: 1 | 2 | 4–6 | 8 | 17   **Rarity:** common

Mica Schist (Metapelite)
Mineralogy: metamorphic rock rich in mica (mon., tert.)
Indications: (SP) detachment, setting boundaries (S) helps face difficulties in a collected and controlled manner (M) helps act rationally and without prejudice even under pressure (B) helps with skin irritations, nervousness, tremors, headaches and vegetative dystonia.
Bib.: 2 | 4   **Rarity:** not always available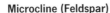

Microcline (Feldspar)
Mineralogy: potassium feldspar (lattice silicate, tric., prim.)
Indications: (SP) pragmatism (S) brings harmony and stability, helps repose in oneself (M) enables sober and realistic deliberation and prudent action (B) stabilises circulation, helps with stomach and intestinal problems.
Bib.: 4–6 | 8 | 19   **Rarity:** scarce ○

Moldavite (Tektite)
Mineralogy: glass formed by meteorite impact (am., tert.)
Indications: (SP) freedom (S) brings unlimited vastness; promotes dreams and memories (M) dissolves attention from strong attachment; promotes the recognition of one being of spiritual origin (B) helps with diseases of the respiratory tract, 'flu and anaemia.
Bib.: 1 | 2 | 4–8 | 12 | 14 | 19   **Rarity:** not always available ○

Mondolite (Iron Quartz-Chalcedony)
Mineralogy: iron quartz on chalcedony (quartz, trig., sec.)
Indications: (SP) alertness (S) strengthens and harmonises; invigorates and dispels tiredness (M) makes alert and endows with quick reflexes (B) stimulates digestion, blood flow and the immune system; helps with interruption and delay of menstruation.
Bib.: 4   **Rarity:** scarce ○

Moonstone, grey (Feldspar)

Mineralogy: grey moonstone (mon./tric., prim.)
Indications: (SP) intuition (S) bestows depth of feeling, helps with sleepwalking (M) makes receptive to inspiration and impulses (B) brings hormonal cycles in harmony with natural rhythms, helps with problems during menstruation, after childbirth and menopause.
Bib.: 1–14 | 17–19   **Rarity:** readily available ○

Moonstone, green (Feldspar)

Mineralogy: green moonstone (mon./tric., prim.)
Indications: (SP) sensitivity (S) helps perceive one's receptivity for moods and situations (M) enables one to talk about (own) feelings (B) regulates the hormonal system during puberty and in menopause, helps with menstrual pains.
Bib.: 2 | 4–6 | 8   **Rarity:** not always available ◐

Moonstone, reddish (Feldspar)

Mineralogy: reddish moonstone (mon./tric., prim.)
Indications: (SP) inspiration (S) helps express and implement feelings (M) broadens the horizon and helps remain realistic at the same time (B) stimulates the hormonal glands, boosts fertility and helps with problems during menstruation and after childbirth.
Bib.: 1–14 | 17 | 18   **Rarity:** readily available ○

Moonstone, white (Feldspar)

Mineralogy: feldspar with swaying light beam (mon./tric., prim.)
Indications: (SP) clairvoyance (S) makes emotional life calm, helps with sleepwalking (M) opens the receptive senses (B) brings hormonal cycles in harmony with natural rhythms, helps with problems during menstruation, after childbirth and menopause.
Bib.: 1–14 | 17–19   **Rarity:** readily available ○

Mookaite (Chert)

Mineralogy: mixture of jasper and opal (trig./am., sec.)
Indications: (SP) experience (S) promotes variety, fun and intense experiences (M) makes flexible, prompts one to envisage many possibilities and always to choose the appropriate one (B) fortifies the spleen, liver, immune system, enhances blood purification and wound healing.
Bib.: 1–6 | 8–14 | 17   **Rarity:** readily available ◐

Moss Agate (Chalcedony)

Mineralogy: chalcedony with green streaks (trig., prim.)
Indications: (SP) liberation (S) frees from heaviness, pressure and strain (M) makes conscious, promotes communication and an alert mind (B) cleanses the tissues, lymph and respiratory tract; helps with cough, colds and stubborn infections and reduces fever.
Bib.: 1–11 | 13 | 14 | 17   **Rarity:** readily available

Moss Agate, pink (Chalcedony)

Mineralogy: chalcedony with brown inclusions (trig., prim.)
Indications: (SP) coming to terms (S) helps overcome revulsion, disgust, resentment (M) dissolves assignment of blame and thoughts of revenge (B) stimulates digestion and excretion; improves activities of the intestine, ameliorates inflammations of the stomach to intestine.
Bib.: 2–6 | 8 | 9 | 11 | 14 | 17   **Rarity:** not always available ○

Moqui Marbles (Limonite Balls)

Mineralogy: limonite balls filled with sand (trig./rhom., sec.)
Indications: (SP) fulfilment of wishes (S) makes active during daytime and improves sleep at night (M) brings wishes and needs to bear (B) promotes regeneration, blood formation and blood flow; activates latent illnesses to enable a cure; fortifies the muscles, intestine and skin.
Bib.: 2 | 4–6 | 8   **Rarity:** not always available ○

Morganite (Beryl)

Mineralogy: beryl containing manganese (ring silicate, hex., prim.)
Indications: (SP) responsibility (S) helps relinquish stress, pressure to perform, pomposity and habit of escaping (M) makes considerate, helps take on responsibility (B) ameliorates problems of the heart and nerves, sense of balance disorders and impotence.
Bib.: 1 | 2 | 4–8 | 11 | 17 | 19   **Rarity:** scarce ○

Muscovite (Mica)

Mineralogy: bright mica (sheet silicate, mon., prim./tert.)
Indications: (SP) protection (S) helps remain relaxed and calm in the face of serious problems, provocations and attacks (M) helps see things clearly and still remain objective (B) helps with problems of stomach, gallbladder, kidneys; trembling and nervousness.
Bib.: 2 | 4–6 | 8   **Rarity:** readily available

Natrolite

Mineralogy: zeolite fibre (lattice silicate, rhom., prim./sec./tert.)
Indications: (SP) wholeness, identity (S) helps trust one's inner voice
(M) promotes an all-embracing way of perceiving and viewing things
(B) regulates the kidneys, thyroid gland and hormone system, fortifies
the intestine, connective tissues, muscles and skin.
Bib.: 2 | 4–6   **Rarity:** scarce ◯

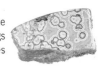

Nephrite 'Jade' (Actinolite)

Mineralogy: interwoven actinolite (chain silicate, mon., tert.)
Indications: (SP) balance (S) protection against external pressure and
aggressiveness; brings inner balance (M) helps with indecision, doubt
and senseless brooding (B) fortifies the kidneys, regulates water balance, and helps with problems of the urinary tract and bladder.
Bib.: 1–6 | 8 | 11–14 | 17 | 19   **Rarity:** readily available ◒

Nickeline (Red Nickel Pebble)

Mineralogy: nickel arsenide (trig., prim.)
Indications: (SP) moderation and circumspection (S) helps with excessive self-destructive lifestyle (M) improves consideration for others
(B) helps with nodes in the tissues, and rashes. **Caution:** very poisonous! Avoid skin contact and internal usage!
Bib.: 4 | 8   **Rarity:** scarce ◯

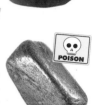

Nickel Quartz

Mineralogy: coarse quartz containing nickel (trig., prim.)
Indications: (SP) revelation, confession (S) makes it easier to express
discord, anger and displeasure (M) helps resolve misunderstandings
and admit mistakes (B) enhances detoxification, helps with dizziness
and balance-related disorders.
Bib.: 4   **Rarity:** scarce ◯

Nuummite

Mineralogy: anthophyllite gedrite schist (amphibole, rhom., tert.)
Indications: (SP) honour, respect (S) reduces tension and stress, aids
deep sleep (M) helps respect oneself and others and fulfil obligations
(B) helps with diseases of the nerves as well as with problems of the
kidneys and ears.
Bib.: 4–6   **Rarity:** rare ◯

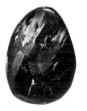

Obsidian

Mineralogy: volcanic glass (silicon dioxide, am., prim.)
Indications: **(SP)** resolution **(S)** rescue remedy for shock, traumas and blockages **(M)** helps integrate one's dark side, activates untapped abilities **(B)** eases pain, tension and constriction of the vessels and enhances blood flow and wound healing.
Bib.: 1–11 | 13 | 14 | 17 | 19   Rarity: common ○

Obsidian 'Gold Obsidian'

Mineralogy: gold iridescent volcanic glass (am., prim.)
Indications: **(SP)** healing **(S)** helps overcome effects of emotional injuries **(M)** helps dispel deep-rooted pessimism **(B)** accelerates healing of injuries, wounds, distortions, bruises and sprains.
Bib.: 2 | 4–6 | 8 | 11 | 13 | 14 | 17 | 19   Rarity: scarce ○

Obsidian 'Midnight Lace Obsidian'

Mineralogy: obsidian with bright and dark patches (am., prim.)
Indications: **(SP)** for new perspective **(S)** eases strong tension and helps free oneself from burdens and painful memories **(M)** helps develop new perspectives **(B)** ameliorates all kinds of pain, helps with shock and enhances blood flow.
Bib.: 4   Rarity: scarce ○

Obsidian 'Mahogany Obsidian'

Mineralogy: brownish black volcanic glass (am., prim.)
Indications: **(SP)** drive **(S)** brings power, initiative and new drive **(M)** dispels dismay caused by insults, disparaging comments and false accusations **(B)** improves blood flow; warms up the limbs; helps stop bleeding and aids wound healing.
Bib.: 1 | 2 | 4–8 | 11 | 13 | 14 | 17   Rarity: readily available

Obsidian 'Silver Obsidian'

Mineralogy: silver iridescent volcanic glass (am., prim.)
Indications: **(SP)** consciousness **(S)** reveals suppressed thoughts and emotions; helps ward off psychic attacks **(M)** improves sense of perception, sharpens senses and intellect **(B)** releases shock on the cellular level and sets stagnant healing processes in motion.
Bib.: 1 | 2 | 4–6 | 8 | 9 | 11 | 13 | 14 | 17   Rarity: scarce

Obsidian 'Smoky Obsidian', 'Apache Tear'

Mineralogy: transparent volcanic glass (am., prim.)
Indications: (SP) eases pain (S) releases emotional pain and helps with fear, panic and shock (M) helps give up belief in misfortune (B) alleviates sprain, strain, back pain as well as general local and intermittent pains.
Bib.: 1–6 | 8 | 9 | 11 | 13 | 14 | 17 | 19   **Rarity:** readily available ◯

Obsidian 'Snowflake Obsidian'

Mineralogy: obsidian with cristobalite (am./tetr., prim.)
Indications: (SP) awakening (S) dispels fear and emotional blockages (M) motivates to spontaneously materialise ideas (B) enhances blood flow even under extreme under-supply ('smoker's leg'), warms up the hands and feet, aids wound healing.
Bib.: 1–11 | 13 | 14 | 17 | 19   **Rarity:** common ◯

Obsidian 'Rainbow Obsidian'

Mineralogy: coloured iridescent volcanic glass (am., prim.)
Indications: (SP) clairvoyance (S) lends the world of perceptions an undreamed-of depth, protects and strengthens at the same time (M) makes open; intensifies perception and sharpens the receptive senses (B) improves blood flow, eases pain and helps with bad eyesight.
Bib.: 1–6 | 8 | 9 | 11 | 13 | 14 | 17 | 19   **Rarity:** not always available ◯

Ocean Chalcedony (Ocean Agate, Ocean Jasper) (Chalcedony)

Mineralogy: spherulitic chalcedony (quartz, trig., prim.)
Indications: (SP) renewal (S) makes positive, able to withstand stress; helps with relaxing sleep (M) helps resolve conflicts (B) aids digestion, warmth, detoxification, regeneration, cell renewal, the immune system and skin; helps with colds, cysts and tumours.
Bib.: 3–6 | 8–11 | 13 | 14 | 17   **Rarity:** not always available ◯

Olivine (Peridote, Chrysolite)

Mineralogy: magnesium iron island silicate (rhom., prim.)
Indications: (SP) independence (S) dissipates anger, rage and guilty conscience (M) helps break away from external influences as well as to admit mistakes (B) strengthens the liver, gallbladder and small intestine; detoxifies and helps with infections, fungi and warts.
Bib.: 1–6 | 8–11 | 13 | 14 | 16   **Rarity:** readily available ◯

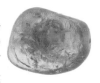

Oncolite (Leopardite)

Mineralogy: limestone sediment with oncoids (trig., sec.)
Indications: (SP) association, common grounds (S) helps participate emotionally and integrate oneself in social structures (M) encourages to share one's talents (B) boosts absorption of nutrients and excretion, fortifies the stomach, intestine, connective tissues and bones.
Bib.: 4   **Rarity:** scarce

Onyx (Chalcedony)

Mineralogy: black chalcedony (trig., prim./sec.)
Indications: (SP) self-assertion (S) boosts self-confidence and sense of responsibility (M) improves rational thinking, logic, control and power of reasoning (B) sharpens sense of hearing, helps with diseases of the inner ear; improves functions of the nerves.
Bib.: 1 | 2 | 4–8 | 14 | 19   **Rarity:** not always available ○

Onyx Marble (Aragonite Calcite)

Mineralogy: banded aragonite calcite (rhom., sec.)
Indications: (SP) rhythmic development, relief (S) makes more relaxed, freer and more sensitive (M) makes flexible; brings harmonious interchange between rest and activity (B) helps with problems of the liver, gallbladder, discs, joints and meniscus (knee).
Bib.: 2 | 4–6 | 8 | 9 | 11 | 17 | 19   **Rarity:** common ○

Oolite (Iron Oolite)

Mineralogy: iron oxide balls in sandstone (rhom./trig., sec.)
Indications: (SP) health consciousness (S) curbs consuming workaholism and enhances regeneration (M) turns attention to health and fitness (B) promotes blood flow and supply of nutrients to the tissues; fortifies the nerves, muscles, intestine and skin.
Bib.: 2 | 4 | 6   **Rarity:** not always available

Oolite Limestone (Roestone, Margarita Stone)

Mineralogy: small spherical limestone rocks (rhom./trig., sec.)
Indications: (SP) purification (S) brings relief in a gentle way, helps sleep through the night (M) frees from nagging and 'brain racking' thoughts (B) reduces fever; detoxifies, cleanses and alleviates headaches induced by the metabolic system.
Bib.: 2 | 4–6 | 8 | 13 | 14 | 16   **Rarity:** not always available ○

Opal 'Andean Opal, colourless'

Mineralogy: colourless common opal (am., prim.)

Indications: (SP) motion in life (S) makes flexible and helps adjust to changing situations (M) brings thoughts, speech and deeds into motion (B) enhances purification of the skin and respiratory tract, stimulates flow of the lymph and excretion.

Bib.: 1 | 2 | 4–6 | 14 | 17   **Rarity:** not always available ⌀

Opal 'Andean Opal, green', 'Chrysopal'

Mineralogy: common opal containing copper (am., prim.)

Indications: (SP) naturalness (S) releases emotions, relieves feeling of unease; lightens mood (M) helps look at the world with amazement and to recognise the miracle of life (B) detoxifies; reduces fever; fortifies the liver and kidneys.

Bib.: 1 | 2 | 4–6 | 8 | 14 | 17   **Rarity:** not always available ⌀

Opal 'Andean Opal, pink', 'Pink Opal'

Mineralogy: common opal containing manganese (am., prim.)

Indications: (SP) warm-heartedness (S) dissipates awkwardness, shame and shyness; enhances perceptive ability and affection (M) makes friendly and open in thoughts and actions (B) helps with heart problems, especially those caused by worrying about the heart.

Bib.: 1 | 2 | 4–6 | 8 | 11 | 14 | 17   **Rarity:** not always available ○

Opal, black, 'Black Opal' (Precious Opal)

Mineralogy: black colourful precious opal (am., prim./sec.)

Indications: (SP) will to live (S) aids a positive disposition to life; helps with anxiety and depression (M) helps easily accept difficulties (B) stimulates intensive cleansing processes, enhances cleansing and excretion; has a regenerative effect after illnesses.

Bib.: 1–7 | 19   **Rarity:** rare ○

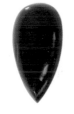

Opal, blue

Mineralogy: blue common opal (am., prim./sec.)

Indications: (SP) sixth sense (S) promotes empathy (M) improves communication, helps understand others and express oneself clearly (B) reduces blood pressure and fever, stimulates water balance, lymph and the kidneys.

Bib.: 2 | 4–6 | 8   **Rarity:** scarce ⌀

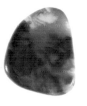

Opal 'Boulder Opal' (Precious Opal)

Mineralogy: precious opal veins in bedrock (opal: am., sec.)
Indications: (SP) humour (S) makes extrovert and helps infect others with one's joy (M) helps survive adverse situations with optimism (B) stimulates the lymph, kidneys and intestine and the supply of nutrients to the cells.
Bib.: 1–9 | 12 | 17 **Rarity:** not always available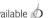

Opal, Cat's Eye

Mineralogy: common opal with glimmer of light (am., prim.)
Indications: (SP) helps comprehend (S) cheers up when despondent, brings hope and optimism (M) allows new views while emphasising the positive aspects (B) stimulates the nerves, brain and sensory organs; improves sense of touch.
Bib.: 2 | 4–6 **Rarity:** rare ○

Opal 'Crystal Opal' (Precious Opal)

Mineralogy: clear, very colourful precious opal (am., prim./sec.)
Indications: (SP) high spirits (S) brings joy, exuberance and a deep feeling of joy (M) inspires imagination, art and poetry, makes clever and creative (B) improves the auto-regulation of the whole organism, keeps healthy and supports all healing processes.
Bib.: 2–9 | 12–14 | 19 **Rarity:** rare

Opal 'Dendritic Opal'

Mineralogy: common opal with dendrites (am., prim./sec.)
Indications: (SP) contact (S) helps remain open and approachable despite bad experiences (M) improves contact with the environment and fellow human beings (B) cleanses, enhances lymph flow and excretion; helps with colds and effects of smoking.
Bib.: 2 | 4 | 6 | 8 **Rarity:** not always available ○

Opal, green

Mineralogy: mixture of opal and nontronite (am./mon., prim.)
Indications: (SP) life perspectives (S) brings quick recovery from exhaustion (M) helps with disorientation and turns attention to fulfilling aspects of life (B) promotes regeneration; fortifies the liver, kidneys and gonads (ovary, testicle).
Bib.: 1 | 2 | 4–6 **Rarity:** scarce ○

Opal 'Honduras-Opal' (Precious Opal)

Mineralogy: ignimbrite with precious opal (opal: am., prim.)
Indications: (SP) hope (S) brings joy in gloomy times and helps overcome crises (M) enables one to focus on the happy moments of life (B) stimulates cleansing and excretion, strengthens the nerves and regeneration, helps with heart problems.
Bib.: 4–6 | 12   Rarity: not always available ◯

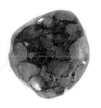

Opal 'Leopard Opal' (Precious Opal)

Mineralogy: small precious opal bubbles in basalt rock (am., prim.)
Indications: (SP) enjoyment (S) intensifies all experiences, deepens emotions and brings comfort during fear and grief (M) aids living in the present (B) enhances growth, supply of nutrients and regulation of metabolism in the cells and tissues.
Bib.: 2 | 4 | 6 | 8   Rarity: scarce ◯

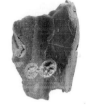

Opal 'Matrix Opal' (Precious Opal)

Mineralogy precious opal in bedrock (opal: am., sec.)
Indications: (SP) living in the present (S) brings joy, luck and peace, helps with stress and anxiety, livens up dreams (M) promotes perception, comprehension and memory (B) boosts digestion and enhances detoxification and excretion.
Bib.: 1–7   Rarity: scarce ◯

Opal 'Milk Opal'

Mineralogy: white common opal (am., prim./sec.)
Indications: (SP) open-mindedness (S) makes open and accommodating; helps accept oneself and others (M) aids communication, exchange and companionship (B) stimulates lymph flow, the kidneys, bladder and the regulation of water balance.
Bib.: 2 | 4–6 | 8 | 14   Rarity: not always available ◯

Opal 'Moss Opal'

Mineralogy: common opal with inclusions (am., prim./sec.)
Indications: (SP) participation (S) helps one better participate in relationships or groups (M) helps approach others without prejudice (B) cleanses the lymph, respiratory tract; helps with coughs and colds; enhances cleansing, digestion and excretion.
Bib.: 2 | 4 | 6 | 8   Rarity: scarce ◯

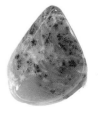

Opal 'Pistachio Opal'

Mineralogy: light green common opal (am., prim.)
Indications: (SP) happiness, joy (S) enhances being happy and enjoying one's life (M) makes sociable, talkative and easy to exchange thoughts and feelings (B) boosts mobility, good for the liver and gallbladder, helps with migraine.
Bib.: 4   Rarity: scarce

Opal 'Prase Opal'

Mineralogy: common opal containing nickel (am., sec.)
Indications: (SP) informality (S) frees from fear, insecurity and feeling of guilt (M) helps unburden one's heart (B) enhances detoxification and cleansing of the body fluids; strengthens the liver and kidneys and helps with rheumatism and gout.
Bib.: 2 | 4–6   Rarity: scarce

Opal 'Seam Opal' (Precious Opal)

Mineralogy: bright precious opal layers in dark matrix (am., prim.)
Indications: (SP) fulfilment (S) helps believe in oneself and allow oneself to have a beautiful life (M) inspires to dare the impossible – and to actually achieve it (B) purifies, improves the flow of the lymph, fortifies the immune system, helps with infections.
Bib.: 4 | 5   Rarity: scarce

Opal 'Water Opal', 'Hyalite'

Mineralogy: crystal-clear common opal (am., prim.)
Indications: (SP) instinct (S) brings clarity in emotions, helps be in the right place at the right time (M) helps recognise and express inner needs (B) enhances water balance and fortifies the eyes, ears, sense of smell and taste.
Bib.: 2 | 4–6 | 8   Rarity: rare

Opal, white, 'Light Opal' (Precious Opal)

Mineralogy: bright colourful precious opal (am., prim./sec.)
Indications: (SP) joie de vivre (S) helps enjoy the beautiful side of life, boosts sensuality and eroticism (M) awakens enthusiasm, imagination and creativity (B) mobilises the lymph, cleanses and helps with coughs and diseases of the respiratory tract.
Bib.: 1–9 | 12–14 | 17 | 19   Rarity: not always available

Opal 'Yowah Nut' (Precious Opal)

Mineralogy: filigree boulder opal (opal: am., sec.)
Indications: (SP) life's dream **(S)** promotes a loving feeling for one's body and earthly existence; stimulates day and night dreaming **(M)** increases power of imagination **(B)** enhances the immune system and self-healing power, helps with very severe illnesses.
Bib.: 2–5   Rarity: scarce ○

Opalite

Mineralogy: rock containing opal (opal: am., sec.)
Indications: (SP) sociability **(S)** helps dissipate fear of physical contact and integrate oneself in communities **(M)** for a good contact with the environment **(B)** enhances cleansing, detoxification and excretion; purifies the connective tissues, intestine and mucous membranes.
Bib.: 2 | 4–6 | 8 | 11 | 14   Rarity: not always available ◐

Ophicalcite (Connemara)

Mineralogy: rock containing calcite, serpentine a.o. (trig./mon., tert.)
Indications: (SP) refreshment, comfort **(S)** helps become optimistic in unpleasant circumstances as well as overcome grief and resignation **(M)** helps think calmly and constructively **(B)** helps with problems of the heart, kidneys, large intestine, liver and gallbladder.
Bib.: 2 | 4   Rarity: scarce ○

Orthoclase, brown (Feldspar)

Mineralogy: brown potassium feldspar (lattice silicate, mon., prim.)
Indications: (SP) intuitive perception **(S)** improves self-perception, helps with fear of failure **(M)** enhances tact and sense of decency as well as respect for societal norms **(B)** helps with indigestion and fortifies the functional tissues of many organs.
Bib.: 2 | 4–6 | 8 | 19   Rarity: not always available ◐

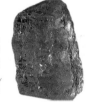

Orthoclase 'Gold Orthoclase' (Feldspar)

Mineralogy: gold yellow potassium feldspar (mon., prim.)
Indications: (SP) perception **(S)** makes optimistic, buoyant and elated **(M)** dissipates anxiety, doubt and distrust; refines the perceptive faculty **(B)** helps with problems of the stomach, heart, constriction of the chest, restlessness and insomnia.
Bib.: 2 | 4–6 | 8 | 14 | 19   Rarity: not always available ○

Orthoclase, white (Feldspar)
Mineralogy: potassium feldspar (lattice silicate, mon., prim.)
Indications: **(SP)** clear-sightedness **(S)** makes more tactful and helps overcome self-centredness **(M)** enhances thinking ability, logic and discernment ability, expands perception **(B)** boosts the pineal gland, harmonises the hormones and nerves, sharpens the senses.
Bib.: 2 | 4–6 | 8 | 19   Rarity: not always available

Pallasite
Mineralogy: iron meteorite with olivine (cub. /rhom., interplanetary)
Indications: **(SP)** insight into primal cause, motivation **(S)** frees from addiction and binding commitments **(M)** urges to discover one's inner world, and to examine the origin, meaning and necessity of one's affairs **(B)** detoxifies and fortifies liver, gallbladder, intestine and muscles.
Bib.: 2 | 4–6 | 8   Rarity: rare ○

Pearl
Mineralogy: radial shelled aragonite (rhom., sec.)
Indications: **(SP)** lends depth of feeling **(S)** helps transform grief, loss and pain **(M)** helps resolve unsolved conflicts **(B)** regulates fluid and hormone balance, good for the eyes, ears, jaw and teeth, helps with migraine.
Bib.: 2 | 4–6 | 8 | 16   Rarity: common ○

Petalite
Mineralogy: lithium aluminium sheet silicate (mon., prim.)
Indications: **(SP)** self-recognition, search for identity **(S)** helps loosen up hardened feelings and face difficulties rather than fleeing **(M)** makes honest and helps come to terms with painful recognitions **(B)** alleviates severe pains and helps with diseases of the heart, nerves and eyes.
Bib.: 2 | 4–6 | 8   Rarity: scarce ○

Petalite, pink
Mineralogy: pink lithium aluminium sheet silicate (mon., prim.)
Indications: **(SP)** self-acceptance, memory **(S)** makes it easier to overcome the past and helps improve relationships **(M)** brings recognition through dedication and commitment **(M)** ameliorates intensive pains, helps with problems of the heart, nerves and eyes.
Bib.: 2 | 4–6 | 8   Rarity: scarce ○

Petrified Wood (opalised)
Mineralogy: Fossilised wood transformed into opal (am./ sec.)
Indications: (SP) for well-being (S) makes open and lively with an unshakeable inner harmony (M) helps see the pleasant, positive side of life (B) gives a healthy appetite, aids digestion, cleansing and excretion.
Bib.: 1–9 | 11–14 | 17   Rarity: not always available

Petrified Wood 'Peanut Wood'
Mineralogy: fossilised wood with teredo boreholes (trig., sec.)
Indications: (SP) contentment (S) brings well-being and makes it easier to accept life the way it is (M) helps use approaching external changes for one's own objectives (B) calms the nerves, helps with overweight caused by poor grounding.
Bib.: 1–7 | 11–14 | 17   Rarity: not always available ○

Petrified Wood (silicified)
Mineralogy: fossilised wood transformed into quartz (trig., sec.)
Indications: (SP) well rooted (S) makes stable and firmly 'rooted' in oneself (M) helps stand with both feet on the firm ground of reality (B) stimulates digestion and metabolism, fortifies the nerves and helps with overweight caused by poor grounding.
Bib.: 1–9 | 11–14 | 17   Rarity: readily available ○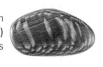

Petrified Palm Wood
Mineralogy: palm wood transformed into quartz (trig., sec.)
Indications: (SP) composure (S) makes emotions flow better and leads them back to a point of calm (M) promotes presence of mind and quick reactions (B) regulates fluid and metabolism in the whole body.
Bib.: 1–8 | 11–14 | 17   Rarity: not always available

Phlogopite (Mica)
Mineralogy: magnesium mica (sheet silicate, mon., tert.)
Indications: (SP) devotion, modesty, protection (S) helps retain innocence and trust (M) reduces excessively high demands (B) eases travel sickness and discomforts caused by inner tension; relaxes the muscles and aids birth.
Bib.: 2 | 4–6 | 8   Rarity: scarce ○

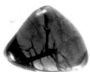

Picasso Marble (Limestone)
Mineralogy: lime rock (calcium carbonate, trig., sec.)
Indications: (SP) abstraction, extracting the essence (S) helps remain faithful to oneself (M) helps recognise the essentials and persevere with turning ideas into deeds (B) enhances calcium metabolism, strengthens the large intestine, connective tissues and bones.
Bib.: 2 | 4 | 16   **Rarity:** readily available ⌀

Piemontite
Mineralogy: manganese epidote (group silicate, mon., tert.)
Indications: (SP) desire, sensuality (S) lends a natural relation to sexuality, enables intimacy and close connection (M) urges one to make the best of every situation (B) boosts the heart, liver, kidneys and fertility, fortifies the sexual organs.
Bib.: 2 | 4   **Rarity:** scarce ○

Piemontite Quartz
Mineralogy: manganese epidote in quartzite (mon./trig., tert.)
Indications: (SP) courage, confidence (S) helps approach others, deal with embarrassing experiences; lends creative sexuality (M) helps express one's needs (B) supports the heart, liver, small intestine, kidneys and regeneration, strengthens the sexual organs.
Bib.: 2 | 4   **Rarity:** readily available ⌀

Pietersite
Mineralogy: tiger's eye and falcon's eye breccia (trig., sec.)
Indications: (SP) change (S) helps in turbulent times; dissipates unpleasant feelings (M) helps digest impressions faster and overcome conflicts (B) eases headaches, nervous diseases, difficulties in breathing, stomach pain and dizziness.
Bib.: 1 | 2 | 4–6 | 8   **Rarity:** not always available ○

Pink Quartz
Mineralogy: pink crystalline quartz (silicon dioxide, trig., prim.)
Indications: (SP) self-development (S) makes lively and cheerful, brings joie de vivre; enhances personal talents (M) helps the unfolding of things one enjoys doing and creates soothing ambience (B) brings well-being, soothes the nerves and overwrought senses.
Bib.: 2 | 4 | 5 | 6 | 8   **Rarity:** rare ⌀

Plasma (Chalcedony)

Mineralogy: green chalcedony (quartz, trig., prim./sec.)

Indications: (SP) for calm **(S)** helps with irritability and aggression; increases staying power **(M)** has a harmonising effect on flighty, disorganised thoughts and actions **(B)** boosts immune reaction and regenerative power; alleviates inflammations.

Bib.: 2 | 4–6 | 8   **Rarity:** scarce ◯

Pop Rocks (Boji's, Pyrite Balls)

Mineralogy: pyrite nodules in limonite coating (cub./rhom., sec.)

Indications: (SP) energy flow **(S)** intensifies emotions and moods **(M)** helps recognise inhibiting patterns **(B)** good for preventive health care; painlessly dissipates mild blockages and makes conscious of more severe ones, promotes cleansing and excretion.

Bib.: 1 | 2 | 4–6 | 8   **Rarity:** not always available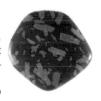

Porphyrite 'Flower Porphyry'

Mineralogy: feldspar in andesite matrix (feldspar: tric., prim.)

Indications: (SP) circumspection **(S)** helps with patience and steadiness at new beginnings **(M)** allows ideas to mature before being put into action; encourages sensible caution **(B)** calms and strengthens the nerves, enhances the senses and keeps the muscles flexible.

Bib.: 1 | 2 | 4–6 | 8   **Rarity:** not always available

Porphyrite with Epidote 'Flower Porphyry'

Mineralogy: epidote in andesite matrix (epidote: mon., tert.)

Indications: (SP) cautiousness **(S)** lends calm and prudent activity, helps with restlessness due to overstimulation **(M)** helps patiently wait to seize the right moment to implement ideas and projects **(B)** promotes regeneration, fortifies the nerves and senses.

Bib.: 1 | 2 | 4–6 | 8   **Rarity:** not always available ◯

Porcellanite 'Eye Porcellanite'

Mineralogy: metamorphic clay (sheet silicate, mon./tric., tert.)

Indications: (SP) ability to differentiate **(S)** helps better perceive emotions **(M)** improves the ability to distinguish between meaning, value and importance **(B)** helps with acne, allergic skin rashes, hyperacidity and chronic tiredness.

Bib.: 2 | 4 | 6 | 8   **Rarity:** scarce ◯

Porcellanite 'Landscape Porcellanite'
Mineralogy: metamorphic clay (sheet silicate, mon./tric., tert.)
Indications: (SP) ability to perform (S) helps express feelings (M) promotes creativity and ability to perform (B) helps with hyperacidity; cleanses the connective tissues, skin, intestine and respiratory tract, enhances excretion and invigorates in cases of chronic fatigue.
Bib.: 2 | 4 | 6 | 8   **Rarity:** scarce ○

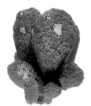

Prase (Quartz)
Mineralogy: crystal quartz with silicate inclusions (trig., tert.)
Indications: (SP) gentleness (S) calms overwrought nerves and makes it easier to resolve conflicts (M) helps people who bear grudges let go of the past (B) eases pain, reduces fever and heals swellings and bruises; helps with problems of the bladder.
Bib.: 1–6 | 8 | 13 | 14 | 16 | 17   **Rarity:** scarce ⌀

Prasiolite Amethyst (Sambesite)
Mineralogy: violet-green crystal quartz (quartz, trig., prim.)
Indications: (SP) authenticity, self-assertion (S) helps stand by one's feelings (M) prompts to defend one's conviction in a determined way (B) regulates breath, the heart and circulation; good for the hair and nails; releases tension and aids excretion.
Bib.: 2 | 4 | 6 | 19   **Rarity:** rare ⌀

Prehnite, green
Mineralogy: calcium aluminium group silicate (rhom., prim./tert.)
Indications: (SP) acceptance (S) makes it easier to accept oneself and others (M) helps accept unpleasant truths and enhances receptive ability (B) aids processing of fat-soluble substances, stimulates fat metabolism and renewal processes.
Bib.: 1 | 2 | 4–6 | 8 | 9 | 14   **Rarity:** not always available

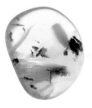

Prehnite, yellow
Mineralogy: calcium aluminium group silicate (rhom., prim./tert.)
Indications: (SP) respect (S) promotes respect for others; helps command acknowledgement (M) dissipates repressive and evasive mechanisms (B) aids processing of fat-soluble substances; stimulates fat metabolism and helps with excess weight.
Bib.: 2 | 4–6 | 8 | 9 | 14   **Rarity:** not always available ○

Printstone (Silt)

Mineralogy: claystone rich in quartz (trig./mon./tric., sec.)
Indications: (SP) feeling of well-being (S) helps restful sleep; invigorates and endows with a deep sense of 'holiday' (M) improves body awareness (B) gently enhances breathing, circulation, digestion and excretion.
Bib.: 2 | 4   **Rarity:** not always available ○

Psilomelane

Mineralogy: manganese oxide (rhom., prim./sec.)
Indications: (SP) promotes composure (S) helps come to terms with negative experiences (M) slows down hasty actions, instils consciousness of saving energy and resources (B) strengthens when under energy-sapping strain; stimulates the intestine, stabilises circulation.
Bib.: 2 | 4–6 | 8   **Rarity:** not always available ⌀

Purpurite

Mineralogy: manganese iron phosphate (rhom., sec.)
Indications: (SP) inspiration (S) helps with tiredness, exhaustion and despondency (M) improves alertness, awareness, concentration and receptive ability (B) gives energy, helps with cardiac insufficiency and functional disorders of the sensory organs.
Bib.: 2 | 4–6 | 8 | 9   **Rarity:** scarce ○

Pyrite (Cluster)

Mineralogy: brass coloured iron sulphide (cub., prim./sec./tert.)
Indications: (SP) self-recognition (S) exposes secrets and suppressed memories (M) makes open, direct and honest; reveals the causes of certain circumstances and illnesses (B) stimulates the liver, intestine, detoxification and excretion.
Bib.: 1 | 2 | 4–6 | 8   **Rarity:** readily available ⌀

Pyrite (Cubes)

Mineralogy: cube-shaped iron sulphide (cub., sec.)
Indications: (SP) serves as a mirror (S) urges perseverance in search for conflict resolution (M) promotes the insight that things that disturb us in others are also present in us (B) clarifies confusing presentations of diseases and brings out the causal symptom.
Bib.: 1 | 2 | 4–6 | 8   **Rarity:** readily available ○

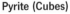

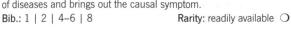

Pyrite (Sun)
Mineralogy: radial iron sulphide (cub., tert.)
Indications: (SP) resolution (S) helps laugh at oneself (M) frees from thoughts fixed on misfortune, misery and anguish (B) alleviates pains such as back pain and problem of the joints etc. and releases cramps and menstrual pains.
Bib.: 1–6 | 8 | 9   Rarity: rare ○

Pyrite Agate
Mineralogy: mixture of chalcedony and pyrite (trig./cub., prim.)
Indications: (SP) purification (S) helps overcome heaviness and strain (M) prompts to tackle unpleasant situations (B) promotes purification and lymph flow, stimulates the liver, improves elimination and accelerates healing processes.
Bib.: 2 | 4–6 | 8   Rarity: not always available ⌀

Pyrope (Garnet)
Mineralogy: magnesium aluminium island silicate (cub., tert.)
Indications: (SP) crisis management; quality of life (S) promotes composure, courage and endurance; dissipates awkwardness; stimulates sexuality (M) supports the striving for improvement (B) enhances blood quality and blood flow; helps with bladder problems.
Bib.: 1–14 | 16 | 17 | 19   Rarity: not always available ⌀

Pyrophyllite
Mineralogy: alkaline aluminium sheet silicate (mon., tert.)
Indications: (SP) self-determination (S) helps set boundaries and to remain alert in confusing situations (M) helps detach oneself from externally imposed obligations (B) helps with hyperacidity, stomach pains and heartburn.
Bib.: 4 | 8   Rarity: scarce ○

Rainbow Basalt (Basalt)
Mineralogy: basalt with cavity fillings (mainly mon./tric., prim.)
Indications: (SP) change (S) gives more room to one's wishes and needs (M) urges to continue step by step on a path recognised as the right one (B) firms up the skin and connective tissues, eases ageing process, helps with indigestion.
Bib.: 4   Rarity: scarce ⌀

Realgar

Mineralogy: red arsenic sulphide (mon., prim./sec./tert.)
Indications: (SP) passion, ecstasy (S) motivates to plunge into intensive experiences and helps recover from them (M) brings awareness of the present moment (B) revitalizes the whole organism, has a fortifying effect on the immunity and helps with draining weakness.
Bib.: 2 | 4–6 | 8   Rarity: scarce ○

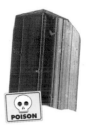

Rhodochrosite

Mineralogy: pink to red manganese carbonate (trig., prim./sec.)
Indications: (SP) activity (S) makes buoyant and cheerful, enhances sexuality and eroticism (M) makes dynamic, active and brings faster results (B) boosts circulation, increases blood pressure and helps with abdominal pains and migraine.
Bib.: 1–9 | 11–14 | 17   Rarity: not always available ○

Rhodolite (Garnet)

Mineralogy: pyrope almandine solid solution (cub., tert.)
Indications: (SP) optimism, zest for life, charisma (S) promotes trust, warm-heartedness, sexuality and sensuality; boosts virility (M) helps face challenges with optimism (B) stimulates circulation and metabolism, improves blood flow.
Bib.: 1–14 | 16 | 17 | 19   Rarity: scarce ○

Rhodonite

Mineralogy: calcium manganese chain silicate (tric., tert.)
Indications: (SP) wound healing (S) promotes forgiveness (M) promotes mutual understanding (B) best stone for injuries, bleeding wounds and insect bites; strengthens muscles, heart and circulation; helps with autoimmune diseases and stomach ulcers.
Bib.: 1–6 | 8–14 | 17 | 18   Rarity: readily available ⊘

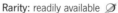

Richterite

Mineralogy: amphibole mineral (chain silicate, mon., prim./tert.)
Indications: (SP) wisdom, foresight (S) gives a good sense of right timing and sequence (M) broadens one's horizons; helps recognise trends early and assess them (B) enhances kidney function and regulates mineral balance.
Bib.: 4–6 | 8 | 9   Rarity: rare ⊘

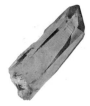

Rose Crystal (Quartz)
Mineralogy: clear quartz with pink hematite coating (trig., prim./tert.)
Indications: **(SP)** sensitivity, love **(S)** awakens and stimulates the power to love, has a comforting and protecting effect **(M)** enhances warm treatment of oneself and others **(B)** protects the heart, enhances blood flow, refines the sense of touch.
Bib.: 4 | 21   **Rarity:** rare

Rose Quartz (Quartz)
Mineralogy: pink-coloured quartz (silicon dioxide, trig., prim.)
Indications: **(SP)** sensitivity **(S)** increases empathy; helps with sexual difficulties **(M)** clearly illuminates personal needs and the desires of others **(B)** harmonises heartbeat and promotes strengthening of sexual organs and fertility.
Bib.: 1–14 | 17–19   **Rarity:** common

Rose Quartz 'Star Rose Quartz' (Quartz)
Mineralogy: rose quartz with light stars (trig., prim.)
Indications: **(SP)** compassion **(S)** makes open, helpful, loving and romantic **(M)** enhances living together in harmony **(B)** helps with diseases of the heart, blood and sexual organs, refines the senses.
Bib.: 1–7 | 11 | 13 | 14 | 17   **Rarity:** scarce

Ruby (Corundum)
Mineralogy: corundum containing chromium (trig., prim./mostly tert.)
Indications: **(SP)** passion, joie de vivre **(S)** promotes bravery, virtue and courage; sexually stimulates **(M)** enhances commitment and performance **(B)** increases fever and blood pressure; stimulates circulation, adrenal glands and sexual organs.
Bib.: 1–9 | 11 | 12 | 14 | 17 | 19   **Rarity:** readily available

Ruby 'Star Ruby' (Corundum)
Mineralogy: ruby with light stars due to rutile fibre (trig., tert.)
Indications: **(SP)** impetus, vigour and motion **(S)** promotes sensuality and sexuality; makes optimistic and cheerful **(M)** helps rightly assess one's strengths **(B)** warms, increases blood flow, stabilises circulation and fortifies the spleen and sexual organs.
Bib.: 1–8 | 11 | 12 14   **Rarity:** scarce

Ruby Disthene

Mineralogy: ruby in disthene coating (trig./tric., tert.)
Indications: (SP) determination, self-realisation (S) joie de vivre, will-power, strength (M) for managing crises, perseverance (B) helps with nervous disease, circulation problems, irregular heartbeat and constriction of the chest.
Bib.: 4–6   Rarity: rare ◯

Ruby Disthene Fuchsite

Mineralogy: ruby in disthene in fuchsite (trig./tric./mon., tert.)
Indications: (SP) protection and self-determination (S) composure; releases tension; relieves pain; promotes good sleep (M) aids coping with problems on one's own (B) helps with paralysis, rheumatism, inflammations, skin diseases, heart and back problems.
Bib.: 4–6 | 8 | 17   Rarity: rare ◯

Ruin Marble (Limestone)

Mineralogy: limestone rock (calcium carbonate, trig., sec.)
Indications: (SP) sense of community (S) fortifies sense of community, faithfulness and unity (M) promotes team work and group consensus (B) stimulates calcium metabolism and fortifies the respiratory tract, large intestine, connective tissues and bones.
Bib.: 2 | 4 | 16   Rarity: not always available ⌀

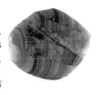

Rutile Quartz, clear

Mineralogy: quartz with few rutile fibres (tetr./trig., prim./tert.)
Indications: (SP) feeling of detachment (S) frees from a feeling of suffocation and lends a feeling of space and of freedom (M) helps develop new life concepts and face the future with optimism (B) helps with allergies, asthma, breathing and heart problems.
Bib.: 1–9 | 11 | 13 | 14 | 17   Rarity: not always available ◯

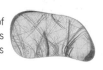

Rutile Quartz, red

Mineralogy: red rutile fibre in quartz (tetr./trig., prim./tert.)
Indications: (SP) greatness, vision (S) helps with sexual problems like impotence and premature ejaculation (M) helps 'think big' and not to undermine one's visions (B) stimulates cell regeneration; helps with constipation and problems of the intestine.
Bib.: 1–9 | 11 | 13 | 14 | 17   Rarity: not always available ⌀

Rutile Quartz, yellow

Mineralogy: yellow rutile fibre in quartz (tetr./trig., prim./tert.)

Indications: (SP) hope, liberation **(S)** lightens mood, frees from unacknowledged fear **(M)** helps liberate oneself from entanglements in situations that apparently cannot be helped **(B)** loosens up cough and helps with chronic bronchitis.

Bib.: 1–9 | 11 | 13 | 14 | 17   **Rarity:** readily available ○

Sand Rose

Mineralogy: gypsum rosette containing sand (trig./mon., sec.)

Indications: (SP) form and structure **(S)** stabilises emotional experience, curbs uncontrolled outbursts **(M)** promotes a fair balance between conflicting wishes and demands **(B)** firms up connective tissues and enhances stability of the bones.

Bib.: 2 | 4–6 | 8   **Rarity:** readily available

Sapphire, blue (Corundum)

Mineralogy: blue corundum (aluminium oxide, trig., prim./tert.)

Indications: (SP) mental faculty, astuteness **(S)** makes imperturbable **(M)** helps gather one's thoughts and focus on a goal with great power **(B)** eases pain, fortifies the nerves, brings down fever and lowers blood pressure.

Bib.: 1 | 2 | 4–9 | 11 | 12 | 14 | 19   **Rarity:** readily available ○

Sapphire, colourless (Corundum)

Mineralogy: colourless corundum (aluminium oxide, trig., prim./tert.)

Indications: (SP) power of discernment, common sense **(S)** enables one to experience the tranquillity of the soul and to draw strength from it **(M)** helps recognise desire and reality and to unify them **(B)** fortifies the brain, nerves and senses, activates the self-healing energy.

Bib.: 1 | 2 | 4–6 | 8 | 19   **Rarity:** scarce ◗

Sapphire, yellow (Corundum)

Mineralogy: yellow corundum (aluminium oxide, trig., prim./tert.)

Indications: (SP) recognition, insight, understanding **(S)** helps feel centred in oneself and feel one's power **(M)** helps recognise the relativity of good and bad luck and to live life meaningfully **(B)** good for coordination, fortifies the nerves, stomach, spleen and pancreas.

Bib.: 1 | 2 | 4–6 | 8 | 19   **Rarity:** scarce ○

Sapphire, pink (Corundum)

Mineralogy: pink corundum (aluminium oxide, trig., prim./tert.)
Indications: (SP) all embracing love **(S)** helps overcome feeling of separation and awakens connection with all things **(M)** enables seeing and speaking from the heart **(B)** warms up, activates the nerves and senses, helps with heart problems.
Bib.: 2 | 4–6 | 19   **Rarity:** scarce ○

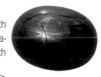

Sapphire, 'Star Sapphire' (Corundum)

Mineralogy: sapphire with light stars due to rutile fibres (trig., tert.)
Indications: (SP) love for truth, composure **(S)** calms and helps with depression and hallucinations **(M)** makes sober and urges examination of the integrity and reliability of oneself and others **(B)** helps with diseases of the intestine, brain and nerves.
Bib.: 1 | 2 | 4–7   **Rarity:** scarce ○

Sard (Chalcedony)

Mineralogy: brown chalcedony (quartz, trig., prim./sec.)
Indications: (SP) heart power **(S)** helps come to terms with disappointments; support with help and advice **(M)** helps master difficult and demanding situations **(B)** improves blood flow of the heart, helps with cardiac insufficiency and irregular heartbeat.
Bib.: 1–6 | 8 | 14 | 16   **Rarity:** not always available ○

Sardonyx (Chalcedony)

Mineralogy: chalcedony/sard/onyx (trig., prim./sec.)
Indications: (SP) sensory perception, virtue **(S)** for honesty and strength of character **(M)** refines perception and aids its understanding **(B)** enhances all the senses, helps ear problems and tinnitus, fortifies the spleen and prevents relapses after illnesses.
Bib.: 1–6 | 8–14 | 16   **Rarity:** not always available ○

Scapolite (Marialite Meionite)

Mineralogy: marialite meionite solid solution (tetr., prim./tert.)
Indications: (SP) carefree **(S)** lightens mood, life-affirming, helps be faithful to oneself **(M)** releases obsession, broadens thought horizons, helps break through 'thought restrictions' **(B)** helps with problems of the kidneys and eyes.
Bib.: 2 | 4 | 6 | 8   **Rarity:** scarce ○

Schalenblende (Sphalerite Wurtzite)
Mineralogy: sphalerite/wurtzite a.o., sulphide (cub./hex./rhom., sec.)
Indications: (SP) upheaval, transformation (S) helps see one through dramatic changes (M) ends futile brooding (B) good for the brain, skin, retina of the eye, sense of smell and taste, prostate and gonads; protects against harmful substances and radiations.
Bib.: 1 | 2 | 4–6 | 8 | 9   **Rarity:** not always available

Scheelite
Mineralogy: calcium wolframite (tetr., prim./tert.)
Indications: (SP) power, ability (S) consolidates one's standpoint and make unassailable (M) brings certainty about one's ability and striving (B) fortifies the brain and nerves, improves tremor, movement disorders and shortness of breath, helps with anorexia.
Bib.: 2 | 4 | 6 | 8   **Rarity:** scarce ○

Scolecite
Mineralogy: fibrous zeolite (lattice silicate, mon., prim./sec.)
Indications: (SP) cohesion, team spirit (S) balanced activity, restful sleep, calms excessive sexual desire (M) helps with positive observation and acceptance of life (B) sharpens hearing; strengthens bones, ears and kidneys.
Bib.: 2 | 4–6 | 8 | 11   **Rarity:** not always available

Serpent Stone (Fossil Foraminifera)
Mineralogy: fossilised foraminifera in clay rock (trig./mon./tric., sec.)
Indications: (SP) contemplation, reflection (S) lends caution to one's involvement with others, or careful withdrawal (M) enhances digestion of life experiences (B) stimulates the stomach, pancreas, intestine, digestion and excretion.
Bib.: 2 | 4   **Rarity:** not always available

Shungite (Black Coal)
Mineralogy: coal in oil shale (hex./mon./tric./am., tert.)
Indications: (SP) achievement (S) helps overcome fear of loss, isolation and material damages (M) enables giving up old habits and destructive thoughts (B) boosts digestion, metabolism and excretion, cleanses the intestine.
Bib.: 4   **Rarity:** readily available

Snow Quartz (Quartzite)
Mineralogy: white quartz (silicon dioxide, trig., prim./tert.)
Indications: (SP) support, caution (S) helps become aware of one's potential and put it to use (M) helps express oneself neutrally and objectively (B) directs energy flow to undersupplied areas, helps with weakness, and strengthens the spine and joints.
Bib.: 2 | 4–6 | 8   **Rarity:** readily available

Sulphur
Mineralogy: sulphur (natural element, rhom., prim./sec.)
Indications: (SP) purification (S) for moodiness and shabby appearance (M) reveals obscurities and hidden thoughts (B) for deep cleansing of the skin, connective tissues and adipose tissues; enhances elimination of heavy metals.
Bib.: 2 | 4–6 | 8   **Rarity:** readily available

Sulphur Quartz
Mineralogy: sulphur-yellow crystal quartz (trig., prim.)
Indications: (SP) purification, clarification (S) helps dissipate anger, listlessness, annoyance and fickleness (M) helps resolve conflicts sensibly and find the cause of all kinds of misery (B) promotes elimination and helps with skin impurities.
Bib.: 4 | 6 | 8   **Rarity:** rare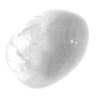

Selenite (Fibrous Gypsum, Satin Spar)
Mineralogy: fibrous calcium sulphate (mon., sec.)
Indications: (SP) shielding, control, strong hold on life (S) calms irritation and hyperactivity; protects against loss of control; helps withdraw (M) for conscious perception and dissolution of personal patterns (B) firms up the tissues and relieves pain.
Bib.: 2 | 4–6 | 8 | 17   **Rarity:** readily available

Selenite (Gypsum Crystal)
Mineralogy: crystalline-clear calcium sulphate (mon., sec.)
Indications: (SP) equanimity, gentleness (S) helps with stimulus satiation, eases stress, brings emotional stability (M) promotes unprejudiced perception (B) calms the nerves, improves movement and helps with motor and coordination disorders.
Bib.: 2 | 4–6 | 8 | 9   **Rarity:** scarce

Selenite (Gypsum)

Mineralogy: flat clear calcium sulphate (mon., sec.)
Indications: **(SP)** grounding, reliability **(S)** protects by making un-influenceable, evokes the feeling of purity and innocence **(M)** helps control oneself and conserve one's energy **(B)** calms the nerves, reduces pain and releases cramps.
Bib.: 2 | 4–6 | 8 | 9   **Rarity:** not always available ◯

Septarian

Mineralogy: calcite in clay nodule (trig./rhom./mon./tric., sec.)
Indications: **(SP)** makes approachable **(S)** helps remain firm in difficult situations without closing down **(M)** dissipates repressive mechanisms **(B)** helps with tumour growth, hyperacidity and intestine and skin diseases.
Bib.: 2 | 4–6 | 8   **Rarity:** readily available

Seraphinite (Clinochlore)

Mineralogy: sheet silicate of the chlorite group (mon., tert.)
Indications: **(SP)** alertness, sociability **(S)** helps dissolve habit of suffering **(M)** resolves conflict; promotes reconciliation and constructive compromise **(B)** strengthens liver and kidneys, detoxifies, stimulates the metabolism, helps with weight loss and promotes a good body feeling.
Bib.: 4–6 | 8 | 12   **Rarity:** not always available 𝄐

Serpentine with Chromite 'Chyta'

Mineralogy: serpentine with chromite (mon./cub., tert.)
Indications: **(SP)** self-determination **(S)** helps shield oneself from external influences **(M)** helps better represent one's interests **(B)** helps with problems of the kidneys, liver, stomach and intestine, especially with alternating diarrhoea and constipation.
Bib.: 1–14 | 17   **Rarity:** not always available 𝄐

Serpentine, precious (Antigorite)

Mineralogy: alkaline magnesium sheet silicate (mon., tert.)
Indications: **(SP)** care **(S)** eases stress and strain; harmonises mood swings **(M)** promotes support and mutual help **(B)** helps with muscle cramps, regulates kidney function, ameliorates hyperacidity and reduces deposits in the vessels.
Bib.: 1–14 | 17 | 19   **Rarity:** not always available ◯

Serpentine 'Silver Eye'
Mineralogy: serpentine with lizardite and chrysotile (trig./rhom., tert.)
Indications: (SP) protection (S) promotes setting boundaries and inner peace, helps dissolve orgasm blockages during sex (M) aids willingness to compromise and curbs quarrelsomeness (B) helps with irregular heartbeat, muscle cramps and menstrual pains.
Bib.: 1–11 | 17 | 19   **Rarity:** readily available ○

Shiva-Lingam (Sandstone, Claystone)
Mineralogy: sediment river debris (trig./mon./tric., sec.)
Indications: (SP) spiritual advancement (S) good for coming to terms with early childhood experiences and other emotional scars (M) helps examine oneself and let go of unnecessary things (B) harmonises and relieves abdominal cramps.
Bib.: 2 | 4 | 6 | 8   **Rarity:** not always available ○

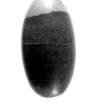

Siderite
Mineralogy: iron carbonate (trig., prim./sec./tert.)
Indications: (SP) firmness (S) lends patience and strength in difficult times; enhances calmness in a harassed and troubled state of mind (M) helps to come out of one's shell and puts a stop to brooding (B) helps with problems of the heart, circulation and iron metabolism.
Bib.: 2 | 4 | 6 | 8   **Rarity:** scarce ○

Smithsonite, blue
Mineralogy: zinc carbonate containing cobalt (trig., sec.)
Indications: (SP) thirst for knowledge, interest (S) makes extroverted, removes shyness; improves sleep (M) promotes intelligence (B) eases diabetes; aids wound healing, immune system and fertility; good for the skin, nerves and restless legs.
Bib.: 2 | 4–6 | 8   **Rarity:** scarce ○

Smithsonite, pink
Mineralogy: zinc carbonate containing manganese (trig., sec.)
Indications: (SP) reconciliation (S) helps master painful experiences (M) brings calm and concentration during changes (B) helps with nervous heart problems, restless legs and diabetes, aids wound healing, immune system and fertility.
Bib.: 2 | 4–6 | 8   **Rarity:** scarce ○

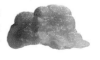

Smoky Quartz (Quartz)

Mineralogy: brown crystal quartz (trig., prim./tert.)
Indications: **(SP)** relaxation **(S)** releases tension and helps with stress **(M)** enhances rational, realistic and pragmatic thought processes **(B)** helps with headaches, tense shoulders and back, relieves pains and strengthens the nerves.
Bib.: 1–14 | 17 | 19 | 21   **Rarity:** readily available ○

Smoky Quartz, dark (Morion) (Quartz)

Mineralogy: dark to black smoky quartz (trig., prim./tert.)
Indications: **(SP)** withstanding exertion **(S)** helps better cope with strain and stress **(M)** makes alert and industrious, helps tackle important things with zeal **(B)** relieves pain and helps with frequent exposure to radiation (e.g. X-rays).
Bib.: 1–10 | 12–14 | 17 | 19 | 21   **Rarity:** not always available ∅

Smoky Quartz with Phantom (Quartz)

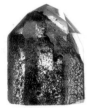

Mineralogy: smoky quartz with obvious growth stubs (trig., prim./tert.)
Indications: **(SP)** willpower **(S)** dissipates fear of failure, defeat or pain **(M)** helps master difficult, depressing situations and to mature in the process **(B)** strengthens the senses and nerves, helps with pain and tense muscles.
Bib.: 1 | 2 | 4–6 | 21   **Rarity:** scarce ∅

Sodalite

Mineralogy: lattice silicate containing sodium (cub., prim./tert.)
Indications: **(SP)** search for truth **(S)** dissipates guilt, helps stand by oneself **(M)** increases consciousness, idealism and the striving for truth **(B)** enhances assimilation of fluids; helps with hoarseness, loss of voice, fever, excess weight and high blood pressure.
Bib.: 1–14 | 17   **Rarity:** readily available ∅

Sunstone (Aventurine Feldspar)

Mineralogy: glittering brown feldspar (lattice silicate, tric., prim.)
Indications: **(SP)** optimism **(S)** life-affirming; dissipates fear, anxiety and depression **(M)** turns attention to personal strengths and the sunny side of life **(B)** harmonises the vegetative nervous system and the interplay of the organs.
Bib.: 1–9 | 11–14 | 19   **Rarity:** readily available ∅

Sonora Sunrise (Cuprite Tenorite Brochantite Chrysocolla)
Mineralogy: mixture of copper minerals (cub./mon., sec.)
Indications: (SP) dignity, beauty (S) helps do away with hurt feelings and remain in harmony inwardly (M) urges to take on responsibility and be meaningfully active (B) ameliorates inflammations, cramps and menstruation pains.
Bib.: 4   Rarity: scarce ○

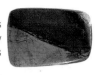

Spanish Olivine
Mineralogy: serpentinised peridotite (mon., tert.)
Indications: (SP) independence, protection (S) brings balance and the feeling of being protected (M) improves concentration and aids self-determination (B) regulates metabolism and the harmonious co-ordination of the internal organs; helps isolate foreign bodies.
Bib.: 4   Rarity: rare ○

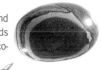

Spessartine (Garnet)
Mineralogy: manganese-aluminium island silicate (cub., tert./ prim.)
Indications: (SP) determination, readiness to help (S) helps with nightmares, depression and sexual problems (M) helps speak out and clarify oppressing and embarrassing 'taboo' subjects (B) fortifies the heart, small intestine (assimilation) and immune system.
Bib.: 1 | 2 | 4 | 6 | 8 | 19   Rarity: scarce ○

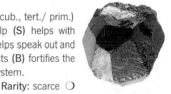

Sphalerite (Zincblende)
Mineralogy: zinc sulphide (cub., prim./sec./tert.)
Indications: (SP) agility, vigour (S) helps with exhaustion, weakness, despondency and fear (M) strengthens power of memory and helps monitor several things simultaneously (B) helps with diabetes and restless legs; good for the brain, skin, immune reaction and fertility.
Bib.: 2 | 4–6 | 8   Rarity: scarce ○

Sphalerite Magnetite in Serpentine
Mineralogy: sphalerite and magnetite in serpentine (cub./mon., tert.)
Indications: (SP) swiftness (S) harmonises inner restlessness and helps fall asleep (M) promotes abstract thinking, concentration and memory (B) improves wound healing, eases diabetes and strengthens the brain, skin and immune reaction.
Bib.: 2 | 4–6 | 8   Rarity: not always available ○

Spinel, black

Mineralogy: magnesium aluminium oxide (cub., prim./tert.)
Indications: (SP) for discipline, duties (S) lends constructive willpower and modesty (M) promotes structure in thinking and perseverance in acting (B) strengthens the muscles, joints and limbs, cleanses the tissues, blood vessels, intestine and skin.
Bib.: 2 | 4–6 | 19   **Rarity:** not always available

Spinel, blue

Mineralogy: magnesium aluminium oxide (cub., prim./tert.)
Indications: (SP) power of imagination (S) helps accept oneself how one is (M) broadens one's mind and enables solving problems from a new perspective (M) fortifies the nerves, kidneys and bladder, ameliorates asthma, allergies and inflammations.
Bib.: 2 | 4–6 | 19   **Rarity:** rare ○

Spinel, purple

Mineralogy: magnesium aluminium oxide (cub., prim./tert.)
Indications: (SP) conviction, attitude (S) brings inner composure, frees from burdensome emotions (M) urges to review one's perceptions and values (B) frees breath, helps with claustrophobic conditions, dizziness and problems of the thyroid gland.
Bib.: 2 | 4–6 | 19   **Rarity:** rare ○

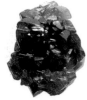

Spinel, red

Mineralogy: magnesium aluminium oxide (cub., prim./tert.)
Indications: (SP) self-assertion (S) lends courage, optimism and life-affirming attitude (M) motivates one not to give up, and enhances perseverance (B) stimulates circulation, strengthens the muscles and revives numb and paralysed limbs.
Bib.: 2 | 4–6 | 8 | 19   **Rarity:** scarce ○

Staurolite

Mineralogy: iron aluminium island silicate (mon., tert.)
Indications: (SP) identity, transformation of one's life (S) helps dissolve fixed patterns (M) helps differentiate between meaningful and senseless things in life (B) promotes a healthy environment for the body fluids; helps with bacterial, viral and fungal infections.
Bib.: 2 | 4–6 | 8   **Rarity:** not always available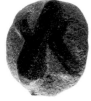

Staurolite Garnet Schist
Mineralogy: staurolite/mica schist/garnet (mon./cub., tert.)
Indications: (SP) fortification, holding one's ground (S) helps cope under strain and to remain composed (M) enables handling what is necessary and completing what is unfinished (B) fortifies nerves, kidneys, circulation, stomach, intestine, gallbladder and immune system.
Bib.: 4 **Rarity:** scarce ○

Steatite (Talc)
Mineralogy: alkaline magnesium sheet silicate (mon., tert.)
Indications: (SP) makes approachable (S) helps overcome fear and excessive defensiveness (M) makes accessible and willing to talk (B) cleanses and releases fatty tissue; helps with excess weight, protects the blood vessels and heart.
Bib.: 2 | 4 | 6 | 8 **Rarity:** readily available

Stichtite
Mineralogy: magnesium chrome carbonate (trig., sec./tert.)
Indications: (SP) gentleness (S) calms overwrought nerves, helps with great distress (M) brings decisiveness in executing necessary measures (B) releases tension in the jaw, helps with teeth-grinding (bruxism) and headaches.
Bib.: 4 | 6 **Rarity:** scarce ○

Stichtite Serpentinite
Mineralogy: stichtite in serpentinite (trig./mon., sec./tert.)
Indications: (SP) peace (S) brings calmness and rejuvenating sleep, eases stress and tension (M) helps make decisions and carry them out (M) releases muscle cramps, helps with teeth-grinding (bruxism), good for the stomach, intestine, liver, gallbladder and kidneys.
Bib.: 4 | 6 **Rarity:** scarce ○

Stilbite
Mineralogy: zeolite leaves (lattice silicate, mon., prim./sec./tert.)
Indications: (SP) gentleness (S) for a calm, relaxed and confident state of mind (M) prompts to follow one's ideas and visions (B) promotes kidney function; fortifies the senses, especially the sense of taste, and helps with sore throat.
Bib.: 2 | 4–6 | 8 **Rarity:** not always available ○

Strawberry Quartz (Quartz)

Mineralogy: pink coloured quartz owing to manganese (trig., prim.)
Indications: (SP) shows cause and effect **(S)** helps not to attach too much importance to oneself; makes witty and humorous **(M)** shows how one personally gives rise to misfortune and failure **(B)** helps with agitation, constriction, and disorders of the heart and circulation.
Bib.: 2 | 4 | 6 | 8   **Rarity:** readily available ⌀

Stromatolite

Mineralogy: sediment formed by diatoms (trig./rhom./tric. a.o., sec.)
Indications: (SP) adaptability **(S)** allows co-operation while still maintaining a firm standpoint **(M)** helps digest experiences and mature through them **(B)** cleanses the intestine and tissues, improves intestinal flora, aids metabolism and excretion.
Bib.: 2 | 4–6 | 8 | 9 | 14 | 17   **Rarity:** not always available ⌀

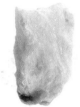

Strontianite

Mineralogy: strontium carbonate (rhom., prim./sec.)
Indications: (SP) esteem **(S)** strengthens self-worth; lightens mood; **(M)** enhances powers of decision-making and outgoingness **(B)** enhances performance and staying power; helps avoid over-exertion; improves bowel movement.
Bib.: 2 | 4 | 6 | 8 | 9   **Rarity:** not always available ⌀

Sugilite

Mineralogy: ring silicate rich in mineral elements (hex., sec./tert.)
Indications: (SP) determination **(S)** helps remain faithful to oneself; helps with fear and paranoia **(M)** gives strength to resolve conflicts without compromise **(B)** helps with pain, nervous problems, dyslexia and disorder of the motor nerves.
Bib.: 1–6 | 8–12 | 14 | 17   **Rarity:** scarce ○

Tangerine Crystal (Quartz)

Mineralogy: clear quartz with hematite coating (trig., prim./tert.)
Indications: (SP) well-being, joy **(S)** makes open-minded and brings hearty friendliness **(M)** awakens interest and promotes creativity **(B)** warms, for good blood flow, boosts digestion, strengthens the muscles and motivates mobility and action.
Bib.: 4 | 5 | 21   **Rarity:** scarce ⌀

Tanzanite (Zoisite)

Mineralogy: blue zoisite (group silicate, rhom., tert.)
Indications: (SP) vocation, orientation (S) helps overcome fear and crises and build up trust (M) helps solve questions related to the meaning of life, and coming to terms with oneself (B) boosts the kidneys, strengthens nerves and has a fortifying and regenerative effect.
Bib.: 2 | 4–6 | 8 | 9 | 19   **Rarity:** rare

Tektite

Mineralogy: glass formed by meteorite impact (am., tert.)
Indications: (SP) letting go (S) helps let go of fear of the future and obsession with money or possessions (M) aids recognition that one is a spiritual being (B) accelerates healing; helps with complaints caused by radiation or infectious diseases.
Bib.: 2 | 4–6 | 8 | 17   **Rarity:** readily available

Thulite (Zoisite)

Mineralogy: manganese zoisite (group silicate, rhom., tert.)
Indications: (SP) pleasure, challenge (S) helps overcome one's limitations; stimulates romance and sexuality (M) helps live out desires, fantasies and needs (B) enhances fertility and regeneration; strengthens the sexual organs.
Bib.: 1–9 | 11–14 | 17   **Rarity:** not always available ○

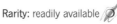

Tiffany Stone (Fluorite Opal Jasper)

Mineralogy: fluorite, opal, jasper mixture (cub./am./trig., sec.)
Indications: (SP) light-hearted freedom (S) intuition, effortlessness, gentleness, relieves extreme tensions (M) for living in the present; makes inventive and objective (B) helps with allergies, lymph blockages, problems of the skin and respiratory tract, infections, cough.
Bib.: 4 | 6 | 8   **Rarity:** rare ○

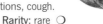

Tiger's Eye (Fibre Quartz)

Mineralogy: yellowish brown fibrous quartz (trig., sec.)
Indications: (SP) gives overview, detachment (S) helps with stress, strain and overwhelming external influences (M) sharpens the senses and helps maintain overview when things are happening fast (B) regulates the adrenal glands; relieves asthma attacks.
Bib.: 1–8 | 12 | 14 | 17 | 19   **Rarity:** common

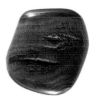

Tiger's Eye with Falcon's Eye (Fibre Quartz)
Mineralogy: falcon's eye transforming into tiger's eye (trig., sec.)
Indications: (SP) enhances composure, detachment (S) helps remain composed in extreme situations (M) enhances quick intellectual grasp and well-thought-out actions (B) relieves pain; regulates the adrenal glands; helps with acute asthma attacks.
Bib.: 1 | 2 | 4–6 | 8 | 14 | 17 | 19   **Rarity:** readily available ⌀

Tiger Iron
Mineralogy: hematite, jasper and tiger's eye rock (trig., tert.)
Indications: (SP) life energy (S) helps overcome difficulties (M) helps carry out pragmatic solutions rapidly and with determination (B) helps with exhaustion, circulation problems and lack of iron and promotes blood formation and oxygen transportation.
Bib.: 1–9 | 11 | 12 | 14 | 17   **Rarity:** readily available ⌀

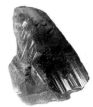

Titanite, green (Sphene)
Mineralogy: green calcium titan island silicate (mon., tert.)
Indications: (SP) integrity (S) dissipates anger, rage and doggedness (M) encourages following one's own path (B) enhances regeneration; strengthens the immune system and helps with stubborn inflammations, bronchitis, sinusitis and root canal infection of the tooth.
Bib.: 2 | 4 | 5 | 6   **Rarity:** scarce ○

Titanite, yellow (Sphene)
Mineralogy: calcium titan island silicate (mon., prim./tert.)
Indications: (SP) integrity (S) promotes self-control, imparts inner greatness and breadth (M) helps struggle through opposition (B) strengthens the stomach and digestion, helps with all dental and gum problems, ameliorates inflammation.
Bib.: 2 | 4 | 5 | 6 | 8 | 9   **Rarity:** scarce ○

Topaz, blue
Mineralogy: aluminium island silicate containing iron (rhom., prim.)
Indications: (SP) self-confidence (S) makes reliable and secure in one's abilities (M) helps gain wisdom from the twists of fate (B) strengthens the nerves, improves digestion, helps with speech disorders and improves the sense of hearing.
Bib.: 1–9 | 11–14 | 16 | 19   **Rarity:** scarce ⌀

Topaz, brown

Min.: aluminium island silicate containing manganese (rhom., prim.)

Indications: (SP) for self-assurance (S) helps deal with experiences so as to gain confidence thereof (M) lends composure through confidence in one's own ability (B) strengthens the nerves, improves digestion and assimilation of nutrients, helps with anorexia.

Bib.: 1–8 | 11–14 | 16   Rarity: scarce ○

Topaz, colourless

Mineralogy: aluminium island silicate (rhom., prim.)

Indications: (SP) self-realisation (S) helps discover one's inner wealth of knowledge and abilities (M) enhances spiritual development; helps clearly recognise one's objectives (B) helps with bad eyesight and eye problems, stimulates metabolism.

Bib.: 1–8 | 11–14 | 16 | 19   Rarity: readily available

Topaz 'Gold Topaz'

Mineralogy: golden topaz containing chromium (rhom., prim.)

Indications: (SP) for self-respect (S) helps become aware of one's uniqueness and to express it (M) lends commitment and willpower (B) helps with nerve problems, digestion and eating disorders (including anorexia); enhances metabolism and fertility in women.

Bib.: 1–8 | 11–14 | 16 | 17 | 19   Rarity: scarce ○

Topaz 'Imperial Topaz'

Mineralogy: pinkish-yellow topaz (rhom., prim.)

Indications: (SP) self-confidence (S) helps present oneself in favourable light; helps with depression (M) helps realise great plans (B) helps with nerve problems, digestion and eating disorders (including anorexia); enhances metabolism and fertility in women.

Bib.: 1–8 | 11–14 | 16 | 17 | 19   Rarity: scarce ○

Topaz, pink

Mineralogy: pink topaz containing phosphorus (rhom., prim.)

Indications: (SP) self-love (S) boosts charisma, warm-heartedness and kind-heartedness as well as a fulfilled emotional life (M) promotes readiness to help and social commitment (B) helps with problems of the nerves, heart and metabolism and with infertility.

Bib.: 4 | 5 | 19   Rarity: scarce

Topaz, yellow
Mineralogy: aluminium island silicate containing chrome (rhom., prim.)
Indications: (SP) self-worth **(S)** promotes self-assurance and consciousness of one's importance **(M)** helps acknowledge one's achievements and actions in life **(B)** stimulates digestion and metabolism; strengthens the stomach, pancreas and small intestine.
Bib.: 2 | 4–6 | 8 | 9 | 13 | 14 | 16 | 19   **Rarity:** scarce ∅

Tourmaline, blue (Indigolite)
Mineralogy: blue tourmaline (boron ring silicate, trig., prim.)
Indications: (SP) faithfulness and ethics **(S)** dissipates grief and blocked emotions **(M)** makes open and tolerant; enhances love for truth and sense of responsibility **(B)** stimulates water balance and excretion through kidneys and bladder; promotes good healing of burns.
Bib.: 1–9 | 11 | 13 | 14 | 17 | 19   **Rarity:** rare ∅

Tourmaline Cat's Eye
Mineralogy: fibrous tourmaline with glimmer of light (trig., prim.)
Indications: (SP) imagination **(S)** stimulates drawing on a rich inner world of images **(M)** brings new perspectives, shows the beauty in everything **(B)** for nerves, senses of perception, detoxification, excretion and joints; effective for the head and respiratory tract.
Bib.: 2 | 4 | 6   **Rarity:** scarce ∅

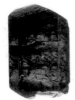

Tourmaline Dravite
Mineralogy: magnesium aluminium tourmaline (trig., prim./tert.)
Indications: (SP) sense of community **(S)** promotes willingness to help, and social commitment **(M)** endows with pragmatic creativity and craft skills **(B)** stimulates regeneration of the cells, tissues and skin; helps with cellulite and healing of scars.
Bib.: 1–8 | 11 | 13 | 14 | 17 | 19   **Rarity:** not always available ∅

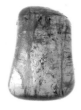

Tourmaline, green (Verdelite)
Mineralogy: green tourmaline (boron ring silicate, trig., prim.)
Indications: (SP) gratitude **(S)** helps see the miracles of life **(M)** promotes interest in fellow human beings and the environment **(B)** detoxifies, strengthens the nerves, heart, intestine, joints and functional tissue (parenchyma); helps with degenerative processes and tumours.
Bib.: 1–6 | 8 | 9 | 13 | 14 | 17 | 19   **Rarity:** not always available ∅

Tourmaline 'Paraiba Tourmaline'
Mineralogy: tourmaline containing copper (boron ring silicate, trig., prim.)
Indications: (SP) love, beauty **(S)** helps experience an all-embracing love for the world and all beings; gives intense dreams **(M)** promotes justice, decision making; clears confusion **(B)** stimulates the hormones, liver, nerves and brain.
Bib.: 2 | 4–6 | 8   Rarity: rare ⌀

Tourmaline, polychrome
Mineralogy: multi-coloured tourmaline (boron ring silicate, trig., prim.)
Indications: (SP) wholeness: brings spirit, soul, mind and body into harmonious unity **(S)** enhances imagination and dreams **(M)** helps recognise and control developments **(B)** harmonises the nerves, metabolism, hormonal glands and immune system.
Bib.: 1–9 | 12 | 17 | 19   Rarity: scarce ⌀

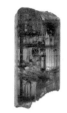

Tourmaline Quartz
Mineralogy: tourmaline needles (schorl) in quartz (trig., prim./tert.)
Indications: (SP) links polarities **(S)** helps resolve inner battles and conflicts **(M)** helps bring contrasts into harmony **(B)** releases tension, spasm and hardening; keeps vital and mobile, promotes purification and excretion; fortifies the nerves.
Bib.: 1–6 | 8 | 14   Rarity: readily available ⌀

Tourmaline, red (Rubellite)
Mineralogy: red tourmaline (boron ring silicate, trig., prim.)
Indications: (SP) liveliness **(S)** makes sociable, lively and lends joy in sexuality **(M)** helps express dedicated commitment to a cause **(B)** strengthens the function of the nerves, blood, spleen, liver, heart and sexual organs.
Bib.: 1–8 | 11 | 13 | 14 | 17 | 19   Rarity: not always available ⌀

Tourmaline Schorl
Mineralogy: black iron aluminium tourmaline (trig., prim./tert.)
Indications: (SP) neutrality **(S)** promotes relaxation, eases stress, protects from external influences, improves sleep **(M)** makes objective, clear, logical and rational **(B)** helps with effects of radiation, pain, tense muscles and feeling of numbness; promotes energetic unblocking of scars.
Bib.: 1–14 | 17–19   Rarity: readily available ⌀

Tourmaline, violet (Apyrite, Siberite)
Mineralogy: violet tourmaline (boron ring silicate, trig., prim.)
Indications: **(SP)** wisdom **(S)** promotes deep peace of mind and helps see life from an optimistic viewpoint **(M)** helps find the right solutions to problems **(B)** harmonises the nervous system and hormonal balance; regulates breathing, the brain and intestines.
Bib.: 2 | 4–6 | 19   Rarity: rare ○

Tourmaline 'Watermelon Tourmaline'
Mineralogy: green tourmaline with a red core (trig., prim.)
Indications: **(SP)** understanding **(S)** promotes love, friendship and security; dispels fear and depression **(M)** helps express one's intentions clearly **(B)** strengthens the heart, promotes regeneration of the nerves, helps with paralysis and multiple sclerosis.
Bib.: 1–8 | 12 | 17 | 19   Rarity: scarce ○

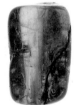

Tourmaline, yellow
Mineralogy: yellow tourmaline (boron ring silicate, trig., prim.)
Indications: **(SP)** happiness **(S)** bestows contentment to life, and confidence in one's abilities **(M)** enhances memory, desire to undertake things and a positive world view **(B)** stimulates the senses, nerves, digestion and metabolism.
Bib.: 2 | 4–6 | 8 | 11 | 19   Rarity: scarce ○

Tree Agate (Chalcedony)
Mineralogy: white chalcedony with green inclusions (trig., prim.)
Indications: **(SP)** for esteem, good reputation **(S)** helps with a feeling of indisposition, restlessness and displeasure **(M)** helps one communicate directly and argue rationally **(B)** helps with after effects of vaccination, effects of earlier illnesses and weak immunity.
Bib.: 4   Rarity: readily available ○

Tree Agate (Quartz)
Mineralogy: white quartz with green inclusions (trig., prim.)
Indications: **(SP)** inner peace, incontestability **(S)** security, stability and perseverance even in unpleasant situations **(M)** helps accept and master challenges **(B)** makes more resistant and enhances immune system, helps in cases of high susceptibility to infections.
Bib.: 1 | 2 | 4 | 6 | 8   Rarity: readily available ○

Tsavorite (Garnet)
Mineralogy: grossular containing chrome and vanadium (cub., tert.)
Indications: **(SP)** uplifted, free **(S)** brings new strength in difficult phases of life **(M)** helps one break through paralysing problems **(B)** detoxifies and helps with inflammation as well as with protracted, chronic and degenerative diseases.
Bib.: 2 | 4–6 | 8 | 19   Rarity: rare ◯

Tsesite (Iron Ore Concrete)
Mineralogy: iron ore with weathered desert varnish (rhom., sec.)
Indications: **(SP)** strength **(S)** stimulates and activates, lends strength and perseverance **(M)** helps energetically achieve one's desires and ideas **(B)** induces inflammations and so loosens energy blockages, fortifies the muscles, boosts blood-building.
Bib.: 4   Rarity: readily available ◯

Tugtupite
Mineralogy: sheet silicate containing sodium (tetr., prim.)
Indications: **(SP)** conviction, understanding **(S)** enhances self-confidence; dissipates feelings of revenge and self-pity **(M)** ends self-doubt and regret; helps learn from mistakes and stand up for one's convictions **(B)** helps with heart and kidney problems.
Bib.: 2 | 4 | 6 | 8   Rarity: rare ◯

Turquoise
Mineralogy: alkaline copper aluminium phosphate (tric., sec.)
Indications: **(SP)** fate **(S)** harmonises, cheers and protects from external influences **(M)** helps recognise causes of happiness and unhappiness and master them **(B)** helps with exhaustion, hyperacidity, rheumatism, gout, stomach pains and cramps.
Bib.: 1–9 | 11–14 | 19   Rarity: not always available ◯

Twisted Quartz (Quartz Gwindel)
Mineralogy: twisted crystal cluster (quartz, trig., tert.)
Indications: **(SP)** orientation, transformation **(S)** clears confusion and uncertainty **(M)** helps cope with complicated situations **(B)** mobilises and controls energy flow, dissipates tension, alleviates cramps, general pain and back pain.
Bib.: 1 | 4 | 6   Rarity: rare ◯

Ulexite

Mineralogy: sodium calcium hydrogen borate (tric., sec.)
Indications: (SP) attention (S) has a restorative and stabilising effect in cases of sudden depression and feelings of faintness (M) helps attentive observation for how things really are (B) strengthens the nerves, helps with nausea and eye problems.
Bib.: 2 | 4–6 | 8   Rarity: not always available ○

Uvarovite (Garnet)

Mineralogy: calcium chrome island silicate (cub., tert.)
Indications: (SP) individuality, independence (S) makes curious and optimistic (M) brings enthusiasm and vigour for one's ideas (B) fortifies the pancreas, aids detoxification and has an anti-inflammatory and fever-enhancing effect (when necessary).
Bib.: 1 | 2 | 4 | 6 | 8 | 19   Rarity: rare ○

Vanadinite

Mineralogy: lead vanadate (hex., sec.)
Indications: (SP) self-conquest (S) helps overcome feelings of desolation, destruction and helplessness (M) helps overcome paralysing issues (B) addresses latent illnesses; helps with stubborn inflammations.
Bib.: 2 | 4–6 | 8   Rarity: not always available ○

Variscite

Mineralogy: hydrous aluminium phosphate (rhom., sec.)
Indications: (SP) cheers up (S) helps with chronic tiredness; eases inner restlessness (M) makes objective and rational; helps express oneself clearly (B) gives energy, alleviates hyperacidity, helps with heartburn, gastritis, stomach ulcers, rheumatism and gout.
Bib.: 1–6 | 8 | 9   Rarity: not always available ○

Verdite (Greenschist)

Mineralogy: rock with fuchsite, albite, chloride, a.o. (mon./tric., tert.)
Indications: (SP) alertness (S) helps perceive external influences; makes stable and able to cope with stress (M) helps take responsibility for one's actions (B) aids de-acidification, cleansing and elimination; strengthens the stomach, liver and intestine.
Bib.: 1 | 2 | 4–6 | 8   Rarity: not always available ○

Vesuvianite, brown (Idocrase)

Mineralogy: group silicate rich in mineral elements (tetr., tert.)

Indications: (SP) strength of character (S) brings steadfastness, helps dissipate anger and displeasure (M) enables resolving conflicts and being faithful to one's principles (B) boosts digestion, promotes convalescence after severe and chronic illnesses.

Bib.: 2 | 4–6 | 8   Rarity: scarce ○

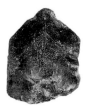

Vesuvianite (Californite)

Mineralogy: rock containing vesuvianite (vesuvian: tetr., tert.)

Indications: (SP) honesty, interest and enquiring mind (S) helps change strong vices and behavioural patterns (M) incites heart-to-heart talk to resolve annoyance and disappointment (B) promotes de-acidification and regeneration; anti-inflammatory.

Bib.: 2 | 4–6 | 8   Rarity: not always available ○

Vesuvianite, green (Idocrase)

Mineralogy: group silicate rich in mineral elements (tetr., tert.)

Indications: (SP) honesty, enquiring mind (S) helps overcome habits and fear (M) helps consciously do away with masks and façades (B) promotes regeneration; strengthens the liver and nerves; de-acidifies; anti-inflammatory.

Bib.: 2 | 4–6 | 8   Rarity: scarce ○

Vesuvianite, purple (Idocrase)

Mineralogy: group silicate rich in mineral elements (tetr., tert.)

Indications: (SP) credibility (S) enables being rooted in one's centre (M) enhances search for meaning and stimulates 'walking one's talk' (B) helps with lack of minerals, regulates the electrolyte balance, protects the skin and mucous membrane.

Bib.: 2 | 4–6 | 8   Rarity: scarce ○

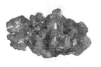

Vivianite

Mineralogy: hydrous iron phosphate (mon., sec.)

Indications: (SP) intensity (S) livens up, frees from buried emotion, makes life intensive and exciting (M) helps with boredom and shakes up rusty relationships (B) de-acidifies; stimulates the liver; helps with weakness and lack of energy.

Bib.: 2 | 4 | 6 | 8   Rarity: rare ○

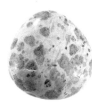

Wollastonite
Mineralogy: calcium chain silicate (tric., prim./tert.)
Indications: (SP) stability and foothold (S) aids resistance against emotional attacks (M) great determination; consolidates personal convictions (B) promotes tissue strength, growth, awareness of the body, posture and coordination of body movements.
Bib.: 2 | 4 | 6 | 8   **Rarity:** scarce ○

Wulfenite (Yellow Lead Ore)
Mineralogy: lead molybdate (tetr., sec.)
Indications: (SP) freedom of movement (S) frees from compulsive restraints (M) helps recognise tensions and patterns determined in upbringing and handle them more freely (B) helps with calluses, dryness, emaciation, muscular atrophy and lithogenesis.
Bib.: 2 | 4 | 6 | 8   **Rarity:** scarce ○

Zircon
Mineralogy: zirconium island silicate (tetr., prim.)
Indications: (SP) purpose of existence (S) helps overcome losses and let go of possessiveness (M) endows with recognition of what belongs to the past and what is really important (B) stimulates the liver, relieves pain, releases cramps and helps with delayed menstruation.
Bib.: 1–6 | 8 | 9 | 11 | 16 | 19   **Rarity:** not always available ○

Zoisite
Mineralogy: calcium aluminium group silicate (rhom., tert.)
Indications: (SP) regeneration, constructiveness (S) enhances regeneration after illnesses or heavy strains (M) helps detach oneself from adaptation to/and external control (B) anti-inflammatory; strengthens regeneration of the cells and tissues.
Bib.: 1–8 | 11 | 13 | 14 | 17 | 19   **Rarity:** readily available ○

Zoisite with Ruby (Anyolite)
Mineralogy: ruby in zoisite matrix (trig./rhom., tert.)
Indications: (SP) dynamic, regeneration (S) revives buried feelings, enhances potency (M) promotes creative commitment (B) de-acidifies, regenerates and enhances fertility; helps with problems of the spleen, prostate, testicles and ovaries.
Bib.: 1–8 | 11 | 13 | 14 | 17   **Rarity:** not always available ○

Search Register

Actinolite: Nephrite Jade

Accumulation Crystal: Clear Quartz 'Accumulation Crystal'

Alum Stone: Alunite

Amulet stone: Agate 'Thunderegg'

Andalusite: Chiastolite

Andean Opal: Opal colourless, Chrysopal, Pink Opal

Angelite: Anhydrite, blue

Antigorite: Serpentine, precious

Anyolite: Zoisite with Ruby

Apache Tear: Obsidian 'Smoky Obsidian'

Aplite: Dalmatian Stone

Apricot Agate: Agate, pink

Apyrite: Tourmaline, violet

Aqualite: Cat's Eye Quartz

Aragonite Calcite: Onyx Marble

Auripigmentum Lime: Eclipse

Aventurine Cordierite: Cordierite, Iolite Sunstone

Aventurine Feldspar: Sunstone

Aztec Stone: Meta-Rhyolite, Dr. Liesegang Stone

Azurite: Eilat Stone

Banded Agate. Agate 'Layered Agate'

Banded Iron Ore: Hematite banded

Beryl: Aquamarine, Emerald, Gold Beryl, Heliodor

Birthing Stones: Biotite Lenses

Dixbite: Deryl, red

Black Coal: Shungite

Black Opal: Opal, black, (Precious Opal)

Blackstone: Gabbro

Blood Agate: Agate, red

Blood Chalcedony: Chalcedony, red

Bloodstone: Heliotrope

Boji's: Pop Rocks, Pyrite Balls

Boulder Opal: Opal 'Boulder Opal'

Drecciated Agate: Agate 'Brecciated Agate'

Brecciated Jasper: Jasper 'Breccia Jasper, Conglomerate

Bridge Crystal: Clear Quartz 'Bridge Crystal'

Brown Coal: Jet (Gagate, Lignite)

Bruneau Jasper: Jasper, beige-brown 'Cappuccino Jasper'

Calcentine: Ammolite (Korite)

Calcite Marble: Marble (Calcite Marble)

Californite: Vesuvianite

Cappuccino Jasper: Jasper, beige-brown

Carnelian Agate: Carnelian banded

Cat's Eye: Chrysoberyl

Cathedral Crystal: Clear Quartz 'Cathedral Crystal'

Celestine in Limestone: Chrysanthemum Stone

Celestite: Celestine

Chalcedony Agate: Chalcedony, blue banded

Channelling Crystal: Clear Quartz 'Channelling Crystal'

Chevron Amethyst: Amethyst Quartz

Chloromelanite: Maw-Sit-Sit

Chrome Chalcedony: Chalcedony 'Chrome Chalcedony'

Chrysoberyl: Alexandrite

Chrysocolla Chalcedony: Gem Silica

Chrysocolla Malachite

Chrysolite: Olivine, Peridote

Chrysopal: Opal 'Andean Opal, green'

Crystal Cluster: Clear Quartz 'Crystal Cluster'

Chyta: Serpentine with Chromite

Cinnabar Opal: Cinnabarite Opal

Cinnabar: Cinnabarite

Citron Chrysoprase: Lemon Chrysoprase

Clay Ironstone: Limonite

Clinochlore: Seraphinite

Cobalt Dolomite: Dolomite

Connemara: Ophicalcite

Copper Chalcedony: Chalcedony 'Copper Chalcedony'

Coral: Agatised Coral

Cuprite Tenorite Brochantite Chrysocolla: Sonora Sunrise

Crazy Lace: Agate 'Crazy Lace'

Crystal Agate: Agate 'Crystal Agate'

Crystal Opal: Opal 'Crystal Opal'

Dendritic Chalcedony: Chalcedony

Dendritic Agate: Agate 'Dendritic Agate'

Desert Rose: Sand Rose

Desert Glas: Libyan Desert Glass

Dichroite: Cordierite (Iolite)

Dolomite Marble: Dolomite, banded, Marble 'Zebra Marble'

Dow Crystal: Clear Quartz 'Dow Crystal'

Dr. Liesegang Stone: Meta-Rhyolite, Aztec Stone

Dravite: Tourmaline Dravite

Dumortierite Quartzite: Aventurine Quartz blue, Blue Quartz

Eclogite: Glaucophane Schist

Elestial: Clear Quartz 'Skeleton Quartz'

Enhydro: Agate 'Water Agate'

Eosite: Dolomite, orange

Etched Crystal: Clear Quartz 'Etched Crystal'

Eye Agate: Agate 'Eye Agate'

Eye Porcellanite: Porcellanite

Faden Quartz: Clear Quartz 'Faden Quartz'

Feldspar: Albite, Amazonite, Labradorite, Moonstone, Orthoclase, Sunstone

Ferro-Enstatite: Bronzite, Hypersthene

Fibre Quartz: Tiger's Eye, Falcon's Eye

Fibrous Gypsum: Selenite (Satin Spar)

Fire Stone: Flint

Fire Agate: Agate 'Fire Agate'

Flame Agate: Agate 'Flame Agate'

Flint coloured: Chert, coloured

Flower Porphyry: Porphyrite, Porphyrite with Epidote

Fluorite Opal Jasper: Tiffany Stone

Foggy Quartz: Girasol Quartz

Fossil Foraminifera: Serpent Stone

Fortification Agate: Agate 'Fortification Agate'

Fuchsite Quartzite: Aventurine Quartz green, Green Quartz

Gabbro: Bronzite Gabbro

Gagate: Jet (Lignite, Brown Coal)

Garnet: Almandine, Andradite, Chrome Grossular, Grossularite, Hessonite, Hydrogrossular, Melanite, Pyrope, Rhodolite, Spessartine, Tsavorite, Uvarovite

Garnet, black: Melanite

Garnet, brown : Andradite, Hessonite, Spessartine

Garnet, green: Chrome Grossular, Grossular, Grossularite, Hydrogrossular, Tsavorite, Uvarovite

Garnet, pink: Grossular, Hydrogrossular, Rhodolite

Garnet, red: Almandine, Pyrope, Rhodolite

Garnet Zircon Quartz: Hilutite

Generator Crystal: Clear Quartz 'Generator Crystal'

Goldstone: Conglomerate

Gold Labradorite: Labradorite 'Gold Labradorite'

Gold Obsidian: Obsidian 'Gold Obsidian'

Gold Orthoclase: Orthoclase 'Gold Orthoclase'

Gold Topaz: Topaz 'Gold Topaz'

Goshenite: Beryl, colourless

Greenschist: Budstone, Verdite

Gypsum: Alabaster, Sandrose, Selenite

Harmony Quartz: Clear Quartz 'Harmony Quartz'

Hawk's Eye: Falcon's Eye

Heavy Spar: Barite

Hematite Quartzite: Aventurine Quartz, orange or red

Herkimer Quartz: Clear Quartz 'Herkimer Quartz'

Honduras-Opal: Opal 'Honduras-Opal'

Honey Calcite: Calcite, honey-coloured

Hyalite: Opal 'Water Opal',

Iceland Spar: Calcite 'Iceland Spar'

Idocrase: Vesuvianite

Imperial Topaz: Topaz 'Imperial Topaz'

Indigolite: Tourmaline, blue

Indigolite Quartz: Blue Quartz

Iolite Sunstone: Cordierite, Aventurine Cordierite

Iolite: Cordierite

Iron Jasper: Jasper with Hematite

Iron Oolite: Oolite

Iron Ore Concrete: Tsesite

Iron Quartz-Chalcedony: Mondolite

Isis Crystal: Clear Quartz 'Isis Crystal'

Ivorite: Dolomite, beige

Ivory Jasper: Jasper, beige

Jade: Jadeite, Lavender Jade, Maw-sit-sit, Nephrite

Jade, black: Jadeite, black

Jadeite, purple: Lavender Jade

Kabamba Stone: Eldarite

Kidney Ore: Hematite

Korite: Ammolite

Kyanite: Disthene, blue

Labradorite Rock: Galaxyite

Lace Agate: Agate 'Lace Agate'

Lamellae Agate: Agate 'Lamellae Agate'

Landscape Porcellanite: Porcellanite

Landscape stone: Kalahari Picture Stone

Laser Quartz: Clear Quartz 'Laser Quartz'

Layered Agate: Agate 'Layered Agate'

Lead glance: Galena

Lemon Calcite: Calcite, yellow

Leopard Opal: Opal 'Leopard Opal'

Leopard stone: Meta-Rhyolite

Leopardite: Oncolite

Light Opal: Opal, white

Lightning Strike Quartz: Clear Quartz 'Lightning Strike Quartz'

Lignite: Jet (Gagate, Brown Coal)

Limestone: Picasso Marble, Ruin Marble

Limonite Balls: Moqui Marbles

Mahogany Obsidian: Obsidian 'Mahogany Obsidian'

Mangano Calcite: Calcite, pink

Manifestation Crystal: Clear Quartz 'Manifestation Crystal'

Margarita Stone: Oolite Limestone

Marialite Meionite: Scapolite

Matrix Opal: Opal 'Matrix Opal'

Metapelite: Mica Schist

Meta-Rhyolite: Eldarite 'Nebula stone'

Meteorite: Iron Nickel Meteorite, Pallasite

Mica: Fuchsite, Lepidolite, Muscovite, Phlogopite

Midnight Lace Obsidian: Obsidian 'Midnight Lace Obsidian'

Milk Opal: Opal 'Milk Opal'

Morion: Smoky Quartz, dark

Moss Opal: Opal 'Moss Opal'

Mother-of-pearl: Abalone

Multi-coloured Feldspar: Feldspar

Muscovite Quartzite: Aventurine Quartz, white

Natural Glass: Libyan Desert Glass

Nebula stone: Eldarite 'Nebula stone'

Needle Quartz: Clear Quartz 'Needle Quartz'

Nickel Magnesite: Lemon Chrysoprase

Ocean Agate: Ocean Chalcedony, Ocean Jasper

Ocean Jasper: Ocean Chalcedony, Ocean Agate

Olenite Quartz: Blue Quartz

Olivine Garnet Rock: Garnet Peridotite

Opal: Girasol Opal

Opalised Wood: Petrified Wood (opalised)

Orange Calcite: Calcite, orange

Orpiment: Auripigmentum

Paua shell: Abalone (Mother-of-pearl)

Paraiba Tourmaline: Tourmaline 'Paraiba Tourmaline'

Peace Agate: Agate, white

Peanut Wood: Petrified Wood

Pectolite, blue: Larimar

Peridote: Olivine, Chrysolite

Petoskey Stone: Agatised Coral

Petrified Wood Agate: Agate 'Petrified Wood Agate'

Phantom Quartz: Clear Quartz 'Phantom Quartz',

Phlogopite Anthophyllite: Hermanov Ball

Picture Jasper: Jasper, brownish-grey

Piemontite Quartzite: Aventurine Quartz, red

Pink Opal: Opal 'Andean Opal, pink'

Pistachio Opal: Opal 'Pistachio Opal'

Poppy Jasper: Jasper 'Poppy Jasper'

Prase Opal: Opal 'Prase Opal'

Precious Opal: Fire Opal, Opal

Purple Chalcedony: Lavender Quartz

Pyrite Balls: Pop Rocks, Boji's

Pyrite Sun: Pyrite (Sun)

Quartz Gwindel: Twisted Quartz

Quartz, containing iron: Citrine

Quartz, iron-free: Citrine

Quartz Gwindel: Twisted Quartz

Quartz, white: Snow Quartz

Quartzite: Aventurine Quartz, Blue Quartz, Green Quartz, Snow Quartz

Rainbow Crystal: Clear Quartz 'Rainbow Crystal'

Rainbow Fluorite: Fluorite, multi-coloured

Rainbow Moonstone: Labradorite, white

Rainbow Obsidian: Obsidian 'Rainbow Obsidian'

Rainforest Stone: Meta-Rhyolite

Receiver Crystal: Clear Quartz 'Receiver Crystal'

Red Nickel Pebble: Nickeline

Rhyolite: Eldarite (Meta-Rhyolite)

Rock Crystal: Clear Quartz (Quartz)

Roestone: Oolite Limestone, Margarita Stone

Rose Chalcedony: Chalcedony, pink

Rubellite: Tourmaline, red

Salt Crystal: Halite, colourless

Salt Stone: Halite

Sambesite: Prasiolite Amethyst

Sandstone: Shiva-Lingam, Claystone

Satin Spar: Fibrous Gypsum, Selenite

Sceptre Quartz: Clear Quartz 'Sceptre Quartz'

Schorl: Tourmaline Schorl

Schiller Quartz: Cat's Eye Quartz

Seam Opal: Opal 'Seam Opal'

Seed Crystal: Clear Quartz 'Seed Crystal'

Self-Healer: Clear Quartz 'Harmony Quartz'

Serpentine: Lizardite

Shaman Dow Crystal: Clear Quartz 'Shaman Dow Crystal'

Siberite: Tourmaline, violet

Silt: Printstone

Silver Eye: Serpentine

Silver Obsidian: Obsidian 'Silver Obsidian'

Silver Topaz: Topaz, colourless

Skeleton Quartz: Clear Quartz 'Skeleton Quartz'

Smoky Obsidian: Obsidian 'Smoky Obsidian'

Snowflake Epidote: Epidote Feldspar

Snowflake Obsidian: Obsidian 'Snowflake Obsidian'

Snakeskin Agate: Agate 'Snakeskin Agate'

Soapstone: Steatite

Sphalerite Wurtzite: Schalenblende

Sphene: Titanite

Spectrolite: Labradorite 'Spectrolite'

Spodumene: Hiddenite, Kunzite

Spotted Lapis: Lapis Lazuli with Calcite

Sprouting Quartz: Clear Quartz 'Sprouting Quartz'

Star Agate: Agate 'Star Agate'

Star Diopside: Diopside

Star Rose Quartz: Rose Quartz (Quartz

Star Ruby: Ruby (Corundum)

Star Sapphire: Sapphire (Corundum)

Sugar Dolomite: Dolomite, white

Syenite Monzonite: Larvikite

Tabular Crystal: Clear Quartz 'Tabular Crystal'

Talc: Steatite

Tantric Twin Crystals: Clear Quartz 'Tantric Twin Crystals'

Tektite, green: Moldavite

Thunderegg: Agate 'Amulet stone'

Tiger's Eye blue: Falcon's Eye

Tiger's Eye Quartz: Gold Quartz

Tourmaline, black: Tourmaline Schorl

Tourmaline, brown: Tourmaline Dravite

Transmitter Crystal: Clear Quartz 'Transmitter Crystal'

Tsavolite: Tsavorite

Tubular Agate: Agate 'Tubular Agate'

Turitella Agate: Jasper 'Turitella Jasper'

Turitella Jasper: Jasper 'Turitella Jasper'

Unakite: Epidote Feldspar

Uruguay Agate: Agate 'Uruguay Agate'

Vanadium Beryl: Beryl

Verdelite: Tourmaline, green

Vulcano Jasper: Jasper 'Vulcano Jasper'

Water Agate: Agate 'Water Agate'

Water Opal: Opal 'Water Opal'

Watermelon Tourmaline: Tourmaline 'Watermelon Tourmaline'

Window Crystal: Clear Quartz 'Window Crystal'

Wood opal: Petrified Wood (opalised)

Vesicular Basalt: Lava

Vulcano Jasper: Jasper 'Vulcano Jasper'

Yellow Lead Ore: Wulfenite

Yowah Nut: Opal 'Yowah Nut'

Zebra Agate: Agate, white/black

Zebra Marble: Marble 'Zebra Marble'

Zeolite : Heulandite, Clinoptilolite, Natrolite, Scolecite, Stilbite

Zincblende: Sphalerite

Zoisite: Tanzanite, Thulite

Picture Credits

Ines Blersch, www.inesblersch.de: All photographs, excluding the following:

Wolfgang Dengler, www.weltimstein.de: Agate Fortification Agate, Agate Flame Agate, Agate Petrified Wood Agate, Agate Crystal Agate, Agate Landscape Agate, Agate Star Agate, Agate Brecciated Agate, Agate Uruguay Agate, Alabaster white, Aragonite brown, Aventurine Quartz red (Piemontite Quartzite), Axinite, Eclipse, Opal Honduras Opal, Opal Seam Opal, Sonora Sunrise

Kazimieras Mizgiris, www.ambergallery.lt: Amber blue, Amber brown, Amber red, Amber black, Amber white

Karola Sieber, www.makrogalerie.de: Agate Zebra Agate, Aegirine, Albite white, Amphibolite, Andalusite, Apatite black, Iris Quartz, Aventurine Quartz blue, Aventurine Quartz white, Basalt, Basalt Lava, Tree Agate (Chalcedony), Clear Quartz Rainbow Quartz, Bronzite Gabbro, Calcite Iceland Spar, Chrome Chalcedony, Citrine, Diamond yellow, Diamond grey, Diamond black, Disthene black, Eilat Stone, Eldarite Kabamba Stone, Fire Opal, Flint black, Girasol Opal, Girasol Quartz, Gold Beryl, Garnet Amphibolite, Grossular green, Grossular pink, Halite blue, Halite orange, Halite purple, Hauyn, Labradorite Gold Labradorite, Magnetite, Moonstone colourless, Nephrite, Nuummite, Midnight Lace Obsidian, Opal white (Precious Opal), Opal Pistachio Opal, Opal Cat's Eye, Orthoclase white, Plasma, Ruby Disthene Fuchsite, Seraphinite, Smithsonite pink, Spinel blue, Spinel black, Topaz Imperial, Topaz pink, Tsesite

Marco Schreier Mineralienhandlung, www.marcoschreier.de: Barite, red

Thanks

My heartfelt thanks go first and foremost to Ute Weigel in Wuppertal, whose request for a wider scope to my book *Crystal Power, Crystal Healing* set the ball rolling. Thus the work on the gemstone guide began in 1993, reaching the first stage after 10 years and now, after 20 years, the second major stage. Above all, my special thanks go to Annette Jakobi for her tireless research efforts, Walter von Holst for all information, comments and corrections related to gem remedies, Dr. Andreas Stucki for the extensive geological information, Bernhard Bruder from EPI for the gemstone analysis and for correction of the mineralogical specifications, as well as the entire team of the 'Neuen Lexikon der Heilsteine' for all the work that has also now formed part of this small book.

In addition, I thank Ines Blersch in Stuttgart for the hard task of photographing 500 gemstones from their best angles, Wolfgang Dengler and Karola Sieber for more first-class pictures, as well as Kazimieras Mizgiris from Vilnius Amber Museum in Lithuania for the special amber pictures. I also thank Fred Hageneder from Dragon Design for the superb feat of transforming this thick bundle of information into a compact pocket guide. Of course, I would also like to heartily thank Andreas Lentz, my publisher, for putting up with the continuously postponed deadlines with such patience.

Over and above, my thanks to all those who made this gemstone guide possible through their contributions and information on current gemstones, healing effects and availability, as well as all those who allowed me to dig into their collections in search of suitable 'photographic models': Franca Bauer, Werner Berger, Harald Bögl, Adriana Breukink, Ruth Degelo, Wolfgang Dei, Beate and Jörg Diederich, Petra Endres, Erwin Engelhardt, Erik Fey, Dagmar Fleck, Manfred Flinzner, Margarete Gebbers, Joachim Goebel, Claire Herrmann, Walter von Holst, Annette and Dieter Jakobi, Angelika Jung, Ava Keller, Peter Kellermeier, Brigitte Krawietz-Rometsch, Tim Lemke, Boris Lessenich, Susanne and Peter Lind, Ursula and Joachim Neumann, Peter Peiner, Jörg Sahlmann, Sabine Schneider-Kühnle, Marco Schreier, Anita Schöpf, Karl-Heinz Schwarz, Isabel Silveira, Andreas Stucki, Kerstin Wagner, Ute Weigel and Sarala Zimper.

Bibliography

[1]   Michael Gienger, *Crystal Power, Crystal Healing*, Cassell, London 1998

[2]   Michael Gienger, *Lexikon der Heilsteine*, Neue Erde, Saarbrücken 2000

[3]   Michael Gienger, *The Healing Crystal First Aid Manual*, Earthdancer/Findhorn Press, Forres 2006

[4]   Michael Gienger, *Das Neue Lexikon der Heilsteine* (subscription), Michael Gienger GmbH, Tübingen 2013

[5]   Gienger/Bruder, *Welcher Heilstein ist das?*, Kosmos, Stuttgart 2009

[6]   Kühni/von Holst, *Enzyklopaedie der Steinheilkunde*, AT Verlag, Aarau 2009

[7]   Barbara Newerla, *Sterne und Steine*, Neue Erde, Saarbrücken 2000

[8]   Kühni/von Holst, *Taschenlexikon der Heilsteine*, AT Verlag, Baden 2004

[9]   Kühni/von Holst, *Gesund durch Heilsteine und Öle*, AT Verlag, Baden 2005

[10] Michael Gienger, *Gemstone Healing*, Earthdancer/Findhorn Press, Forres 2014

[11] Gienger/Maier, *Heilsteine der Organuhr*, Neue Erde, Saarbrücken 2007

[12] Michael Gienger, *Ein Stein für jeden Anlass*, Neue Erde, Saarbrücken 2013

[13] Gienger/Goebel, *Gem Water*, Earthdancer/Findhorn Press, Forres 2008

[14] Gienger/Goebel, *Wassersteine*, Neue Erde, Saarbrücken 2007

[15] Gienger/Glaser, *Salz*, Neue Erde, Saarbrücken 2003

[16] Michael Gienger, *Die Heilsteine der Hildegard von Bingen*, Neue Erde, Saarbrücken 2004

[17] Michael Gienger et al., *Edelstein-Massagen*, Neue Erde, Saarbrücken 2004

[18] Michael Gienger, *Twelve Essential Healing Crystals*, Neue Erde, Earthdancer/Findhorn Press, Forres 2014

[19] Bernhard Bruder, *Geschoente Steine*, Neue Erde, Saarbrücken 2005

[20] Audronė Ilgevičienė, *Bernstein – Stein des Meeres, des Lichtes und der Sonne*, Neue Erde, Saarbrücken 2009

[21] Isabel Silveira, *Quartz Crystals*, Earthdancer/Findhorn Press, Forres 2009

The numbers refer to the bibliography indicated for the individual gemstone entries of this guide.

Addresses

Michael Gienger GmbH
Gemstone consultation services, seminars on gem remedy and litestyle arrangement
www.michael-gienger.de

Das Neue Lexikon der Heilsteine
The most current and most comprehensive information on healing crystals
www.lexikon-der-heilsteine.de

Fair Trade Minerals & Gems e.V.
Association for the promotion of fairness and humanitarianism in mineral and gemstone trade worldwide
www.fairtrademinerals.de

Edelstein-Massagen
Information and contact addresses for gemstone massages
www.edelstein-massagen.de

Die Steinheilkunde
Article, Information and the latest developments in the field of gem remedy
www.steinheilkunde.de

Steinheilkunde e.V.
Gem remedy research, public relations, consumer protection
www.steinheilkunde ev.de

Cairn Elen Steinheilkunde-Netzwerk
Gemstone consultation services, seminars and training on gem remedies
www.steinheilkunde-netzwerk.de

Cairn Elen Lebensschulen
Gemstone consultation services, seminars and training in gem remedies
www.cairn-elen.de
www.cairn-elen-annette-jakobi.de
www.cairn-elen-dagmar-fleck.de

EPI – Institut für Edelstein Prüfung
Gemstone verification institute; issues authenticity seal to professional traders dealing in verified gemstones (GKS seal).
www.epigem.de

Freiraum Media
Lectures and seminars by Michael Gienger on DVD
www.freiraum-media.com

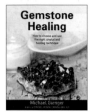

Aquamarine helps against allergies, amber improves sleep and amethyst promotes mental clarity. But what's the best way to use crystals? This practical book is the first to explain the complete range of applications.

Michael Gienger
Gemstone Healing
How to choose and use the right crystal
and healing technique
Paperback, full colour throughout, 104 pages
ISBN 978-1-84409-646-6

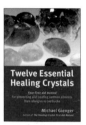

Twelve Essential Healing Crystals embraces many applications. Although describing only twelve stones, the breadth of its scope resembles a home pharmacy. From allergies to toothache, you will find the right stone for every sort of application. This handy little book offers you the essence of our modern knowledge of healing stones.

Michael Gienger
Twelve Essential Healing Crystals
Your first aid manual for preventing and treating
common ailments from allergies to toothache
Paperback, full colour throughout, 64 pages
ISBN 978-1-84409-642-8

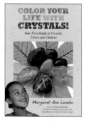

Tapping into children's seemingly inherent love of rocks, this accessible introduction to gemology provides youngsters with a base understanding of crystal qualities, the power of colours, and the metaphysical importance of positive thinking. Divided into seven sections, each chakra is explored and visualisation exercises are included in order to experience the chakra's energy.

Margaret Ann Lembo
Color Your Life With Crystals
Your first guide to crystals, colors and chakras
Paperback, full colour throughout, 112 pages
ISBN 978-1-84409-605-3

Powerful yet concise, this revolutionary guide summarises the Hawaiian ritual of forgiveness and offers methods for immediately creating positive effects in everyday life. Ho'oponopono consists of four consecutive magic sentences: 'I am sorry. Please forgive me. I love you. Thank you.' By addressing issues using these simple sentences, we get to own our feelings and accept unconditional love, so that unhealthy situations transform into favourable experiences.

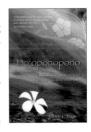

Ulrich Emil Duprée
Ho'oponopono
the Hawaiian forgiveness ritual
as the key to your life's fulfilment
Paperback, full colour throughout, 96 pages
ISBN 978-1-84409-597-1

This is an easy-to-use A–Z guide for treating many common ailments and illnesses with the help of crystal therapy. It includes a comprehensive colour appendix with photographs and short descriptions of each gemstone recommended.

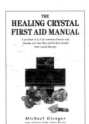

Michael Gienger
The Healing Crystal First Aid Manual
A practical A to Z of common ailments and illnesses
and how they can be best treated with crystal therapy.
Paperback, with 16 colour plates, 288 pages
ISBN 978-1-84409-084-6

There are two types of angels: those with wings, and those with leaves. For thousands of years, those seeking advice or wanting to give thanks to Mother Nature have walked the ancient paths into the sacred grove. Because today sacred groves have become scarcer, and venerable old trees in tranquil spots are hard to find when we need them, we are pleased to present this tree oracle to bring the tree angels closer to us all once more.

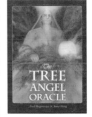

Fred Hageneder, Anne Heng
The Tree Angel Oracle
36 colour cards (95 x 133 mm) plus book, 112 pages
ISBN 978-1-84409-078-5

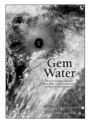

Adding crystals to water is both visually appealing and healthy. It is a known fact that water carries mineral information and Gem Water provides effective remedies, acting quickly on a physical level. It is similar and complementary to wearing crystals, but the effects are not necessarily the same.

Gem Water needs to be prepared and applied with care; this book explains everything you need to know to get started!

Michael Gienger, Joachim Goebel
Gem Water
How to prepare and use more than
130 crystal waters for therapeutic treatments
Paperback, full colour throughout, 96 pages
ISBN 978-1-84409-131-7

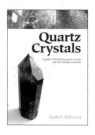

This visually impressive book brings the reader up close to the beauty and diversity of the quartz crystal family. Its unique and concise presentation allows the reader to quickly and easily identify an array of quartz crystals and become familiar with their distinctive features and energetic properties.

Isabel Silveira
Quartz Crystals
A guide to identifying quartz crystals
and their healing properties
Paperback, full colour throughout, 80 pages
ISBN 978-1-84409-148-5

This useful little guidebook provides everything you need to know about cleansing crystals – both the well-known and the less well-known methods – clearly explaining which method is best for each purpose, whether for discharging or charging, cleansing on an external or energetic level, or eliminating foreign information.

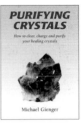

Michael Gienger
Purifying Crystals
How to clear, charge and purify your healing crystals
Paperback, full colour throughout, 64 pages
ISBN 978-1-84409-147-8

The Complete Guide to Manifesting with Crystals shows you how to use crystals to create the life you want. Work with crystal energy to focus your intentions, manifest your goals, support your soul journey and attract abundance into your life. Relationships, health, well-being, career – all can be improved with crystal awareness. Let crystals light your path clear!

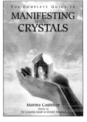

Marina Costelloe
The Complete Guide to Manifesting with Crystals
Paperback, black and white, 80 pages
ISBN 978-1-84409-169-0

For further information and book catalogue contact:
Findhorn Press Ltd., 117–121 High Street, Forres IV36 3TE, Scotland.
Earthdancer Books is an Imprint of Findhorn Press.
tel +44 (0)1309-690582 · fax +44 (0)131 777 2711 · info@findhornpress.com
www.earthdancer.co.uk · www.findhornpress.com

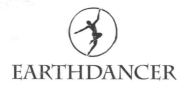

EARTHDANCER

A FINDHORN PRESS IMPRINT